Extracranial/Intracranial Anastomosis

General Editor, Wolfe Surgical Atlases:
William F. Walker, DSc, ChM, FRCS (Edin. and England), FRS (Edin.).

Single Surgical Procedures 20

A Colour Atlas of Extracranial/Intracranial Anastomosis

John S. P. Lumley
MS, MBBS (London), FRCS(Eng), MRCS(Eng), LRCP (London), FGA
Professor of Vascular Surgery,
Surgical Professorial Unit,
St Bartholomew's Hospital, London

Wolfe Medical Publications Ltd

Published by Wolfe Medical Publications Ltd, 1984
Printed by Royal Smeets Offset b.v., Weert, Netherlands
ISBN 0 7234 1012 7

ISS 0264-8695

This book is one of the titles in the series of Wolfe Single Surgical Procedures, a series which will eventually cover some 200 titles.

If you wish to be kept informed of new additions to the series and receive details of our other titles, please write to Wolfe Medical Publications Ltd, Wolfe House, 3 Conway Street, London W1P 6HE.

A few of the other titles in print and in preparation in the Single Surgical Procedures series

Parotidectomy
Traditional Menisectomy
Inguinal Hernias & Hydroceles in Infants and Children
Surgery for Pancreatic & Associated Carcinomata
Subtotal Thyroidectomy
Boari Bladder-Flap Procedure
Treatment of Carpal Tunnel Syndrome
Anterior Resection of Rectum
Seromyotomy for Chronic Duodenal Ulcer
Renal Transplant
Carpal Tunnel Syndrome
Surgery for Undescended Testes
Internal Carotid Artery Surgery
Resection of Aortic Aneurysm
Modified Radical Mastectomy
Discogram Surgery – Lumbar Disc
Total Gastrectomy
Ileo-Rectal Anastomosis
Pre-Prosthetic Oral Surgery
Techniques of Nerve Grafting and Repair
Surgery for Dupuytren's Contracture
Athrodesis of the Ankle
Surgery for Congenital Dislocation of the Hip
Common Operations of the Foot
Femoral and Tibial Osteotomy
Maxillo-Facial Traumatology
Surgery for Chondromalacia Patellae
Stabilisation for Extensive Spinal Injury
Spondylolisthesis
Laminectomy
Gall Bladder Cholecystectomy
Repair of Prolapsed Rectum
Proctocolectomy
Resection of Oesophagus
Splenectomy
Thyroid Lobectomy
Hirschprung's Disease
Anterior Nephrectomy
Bladder Augmentation
Caecocystoplasty
Hiatus Hernia
Total Gastrectomy
Billroth 1 Gastrectomy
Billroth 2 Gastrectomy
Abdominal Incisions
Thoracotomy
Chronic Pancreatitis Operation
Surgery for Strictures in Common Bile Duct
Biliary Enteric Anastomosis
Partial Hepatectomy
Splenectomy
Right Hemicolectomy
Appendicectomy
Incisional Hernia
Lung Lobectomy
Lung Removal
Gastric Reconstruction
Surgery for Lymphoedema
Liver Transplant
Pancreas Transplant
Dialysis Techniques
Surgery for Thoracic Outlet
Haemorrhoids
Abdominoperineal Resection of Rectum
Rectosigmoid Resection
Non-resectional Surgery for Multiple Bowel Stenosis
Surgery for Anorectal Incontinence
Craniotomy
Parathyroidectomy
Arterial Injuries
Arterial Bypass Grafts in Leg
Visceral Vascular Occlusion
Varicose Veins Surgery under Local Anaesthesia
Aortofemoral Bypass
Aortoilac Disobliteration
Technique of Small Vessel Repair
Technique of Nerve Grafting and Repair
Microsurgery Techniques
Reimplantation of Ureters
Pyloric Stenosis in Children
Cleft Palate Surgery
Anorectal Malformation
Amputations of the Lower Limb
Anterolateral Decompression
Spinal Fusion
Scoliosis
Spinal Fusion for Low Back Pain
Anterior Fusion of Cervical Spine
Recurrent Dislocation of Shoulder
Joint Replacement of Elbow
Joint Replacement of Wrist and Hand
Operative Fixation of Fractures of the Forearm
Joint Replacement at the Hip
Joint Replacement at the Knee
Arthrodesis of the Knee
Triple Arthrodesis
Amputations of the Upper Limb and Hand
Plastering Techniques
Operations for Peripheral Nerve
Compression Syndromes
Techniques of Tendon Transfer in the Upper Limb
Arthrodesis of the Wrist
Reconstructive Procedures of the Thumb
Flexor Tendon Repair and Grafting
Minor Operative Procedures
Technique of Arthroscopy of the Knee
Management of Fresh Ligamentous Injuries of the Knee

Contents

Acknowledgements

I wish to thank Julie A. Dorrington and the Department of Medical Illustration, St Bartholomew's Hospital, London for all their help during the preparation of this book.

Introduction

Over 10 per cent of deaths in developed countries are caused by stroke; this together with the devastating effects of stroke morbidity, both on patients and their associates, emphasises the need for the continual search for effective stroke prophylaxis. The transient ischaemic attack (TIA), for many decades, has been the clinical indicator of cerebrovascular disease. However, the widely diverse figures on the natural history of the symptom emphasises the lack of consistency in its diagnosis. Similarly the presence of cerebral infarction, as demonstrated on CAT scan, in a number of these patients indicates the need for a more sophisticated classification. It is hoped that the wider application of digital angiography and newer screening techniques will be of value in this respect.

The carotid bifurcation is the most common site for atheromatous disease and carotid endarterectomy is the procedure most widely practised in surgical stroke prophylaxis. It is complicated by a high incidence of reflexogenic changes, but the operative morbidity and mortality are mainly related to technical problems and to patients with severe bilateral internal carotid artery stenosis. The latter effect is possibly caused by acute reperfusion of a poorly perfused cerebrovascular bed. Further research into these operative problems must parallel studies into the natural history of the disease.

Carotid artery disease, however, is not always amenable to surgery of the carotid bifurcation. Occlusion of the internal carotid artery and distal disease, at the level of the syphon, as well as disease of the middle cerebral artery, are not amenable to conventional vascular surgical techniques. Donaghy and Yasargil introduced the operation of superficial temporal to middle cerebral artery bypass which provided a means of treating this distal disease in symptomatic patients.

Although the procedure did not gain immediate application, because it required the dual training in neurosurgery and microvascular techniques, it is now widely practised and a number of centres have series of many hundreds of patients. The morbidity and mortality of transcranial bypass is much lower than direct carotid bifurcation surgery and long-term results show a prophylactic benefit. Patency is remarkably high, this being probably related to the low incidence of small vessel cerebral atheroma and the high pressure gradient across the anastomosis in the patients requiring the procedure. Initial flow in the bypass may be only 20 ml to 30 ml, but this provides an element of protection to potentially ischaemic brain tissue; it is a common finding that the superficial temporal artery undergoes a two-fold or three-fold enlargement over the subsequent months.

Additional rare indications for the procedure are anomalies of the Circle of Willis, slowly growing tumours around the base of the skull and patients undergoing internal carotid artery ligation for giant aneurysms. Identification of patients in need of transcranial bypass, like carotid endarterectomy, at present is mainly based on transient ischaemic attacks and milder degrees of established stroke.

Preparing the patient

1 The patient is anaesthetised with endotracheal intubation. The tube is strapped into position and the patient's eyes are covered with micropore tape. The hips are in a lateral position, the shoulders slightly oblique, and the head in a true lateral (maintained in position by a deflated bean bag).

1

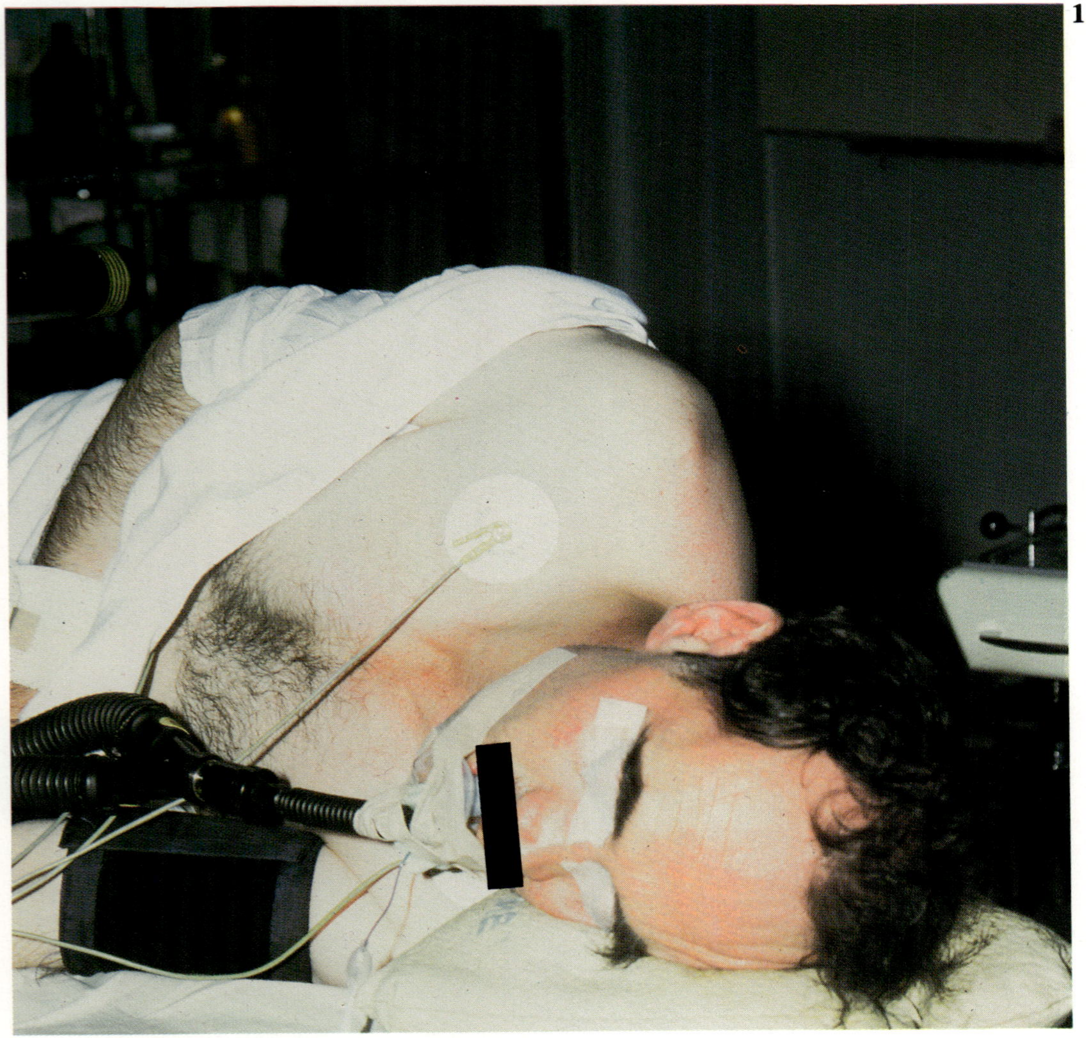

2

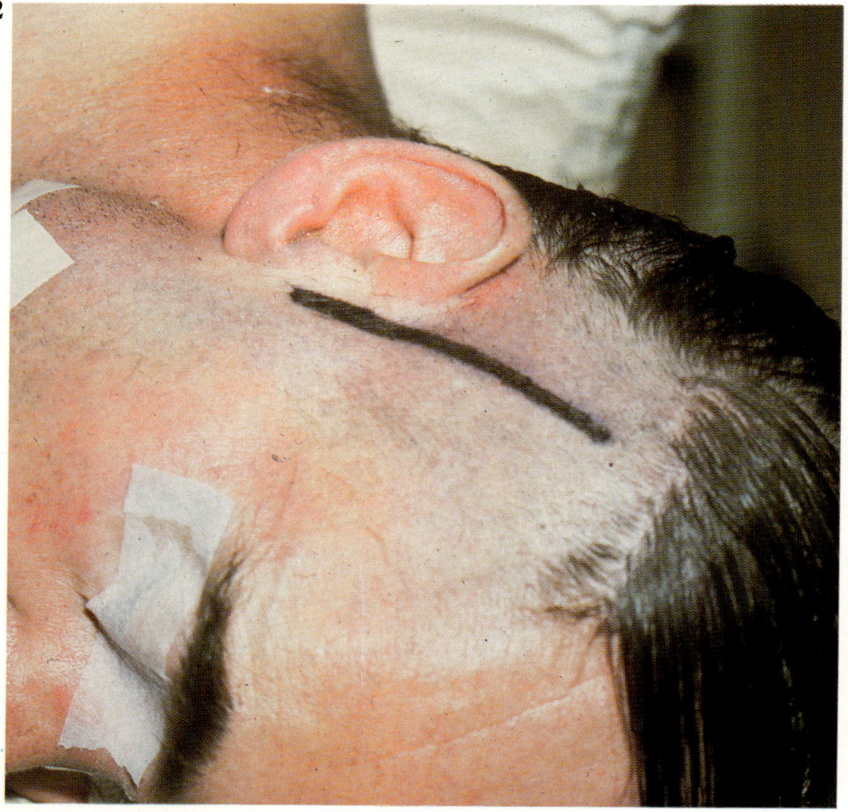

2 The scalp marking indicates the position of the posterior branch of the superficial temporal artery. Hair has been clipped and dry shaved from the temporal region and the uncut hair has been soaped and brushed away from the operating field.

3

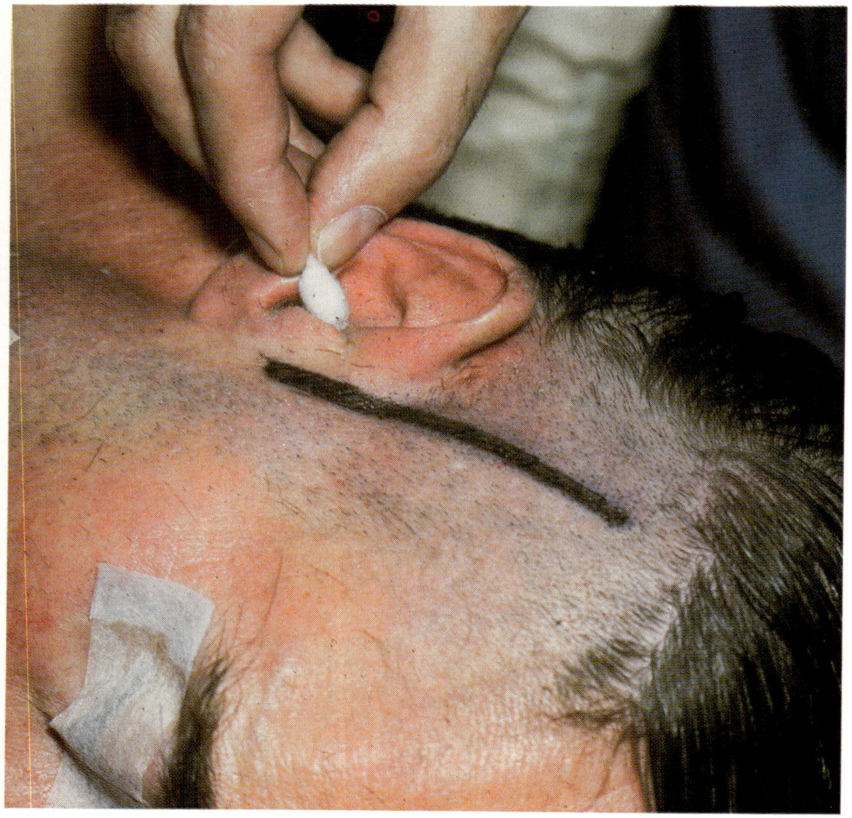

3 Cotton wool placed in external auditory meatus to absorb excess skin preparation fluid.

4 Microscope brought into position over the proposed site of anastomosis and focused on to the scalp. The foot control is used to position the body of the microscope at its maximum height; this allows subsequent lowering to focus on the surface of the brain without additional adjustment on the main column. The surgeon and assistant check the eye-piece adjustments and seating arrangements to ensure they are optimal for subsequent microsurgery. All locking screws, except the one on the main stand, controlling horizontal movement, are tightened and the microscope swung out of the operating field. The third position on the beam splitter of the microscope in this case is given over to a camera, but a viewing arm or television camera can be used depending on local requirements. No attempt has been made to sterilise the instrument or cover it with sterile drapes; instead it has been cleaned carefully and all dust removed: it being managed in a similar fashion to an operating light. All personnel must ensure that no sterile towels, equipment or parts of members of the scrubbed team come into contact with the unsterile surface.

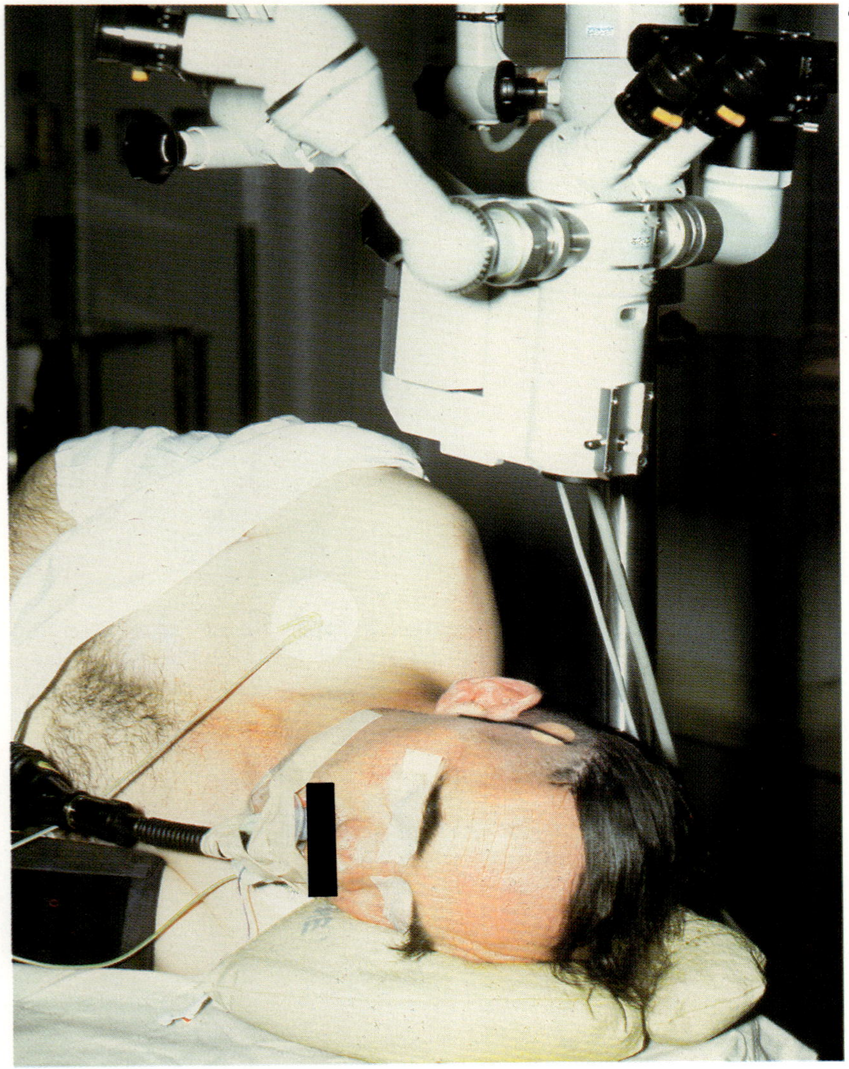

4

Skin preparation

5 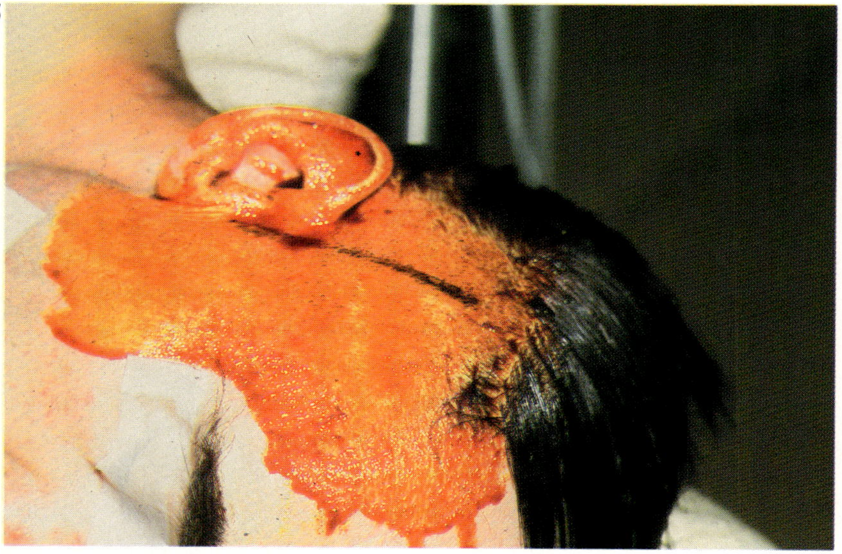

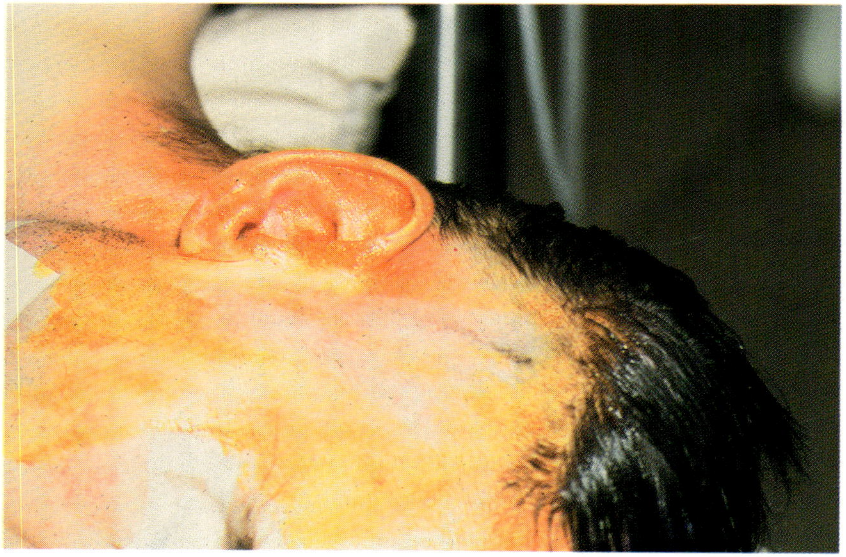 6

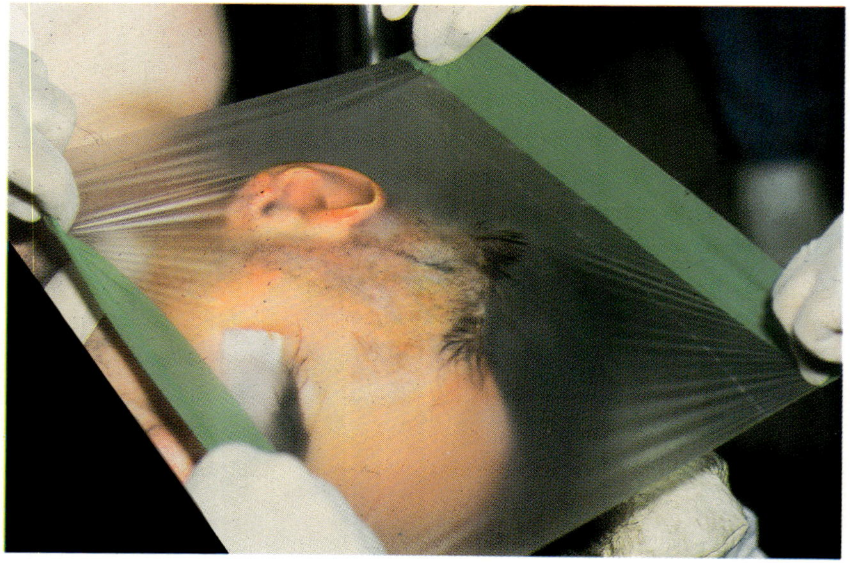 7

5 The skin is prepared with Betadine in spirit. Some excess fluid has passed into the ear. Care is taken that no fluid runs into the eye; such an occurrence requires immediate cleaning and washing of the eye and further skin preparation.

6 Excess skin preparation fluid has been removed with a dry swab.

7 Steridrape is applied to the dried skin, serving to isolate the operating field from the patient's hair.

Application of towels

8 Three of the tetra towels are in position. The posterior clip enters the patient's scalp to stabilise the towels, but care must be taken not to traumatise the patient's face with subsequent clips.

8

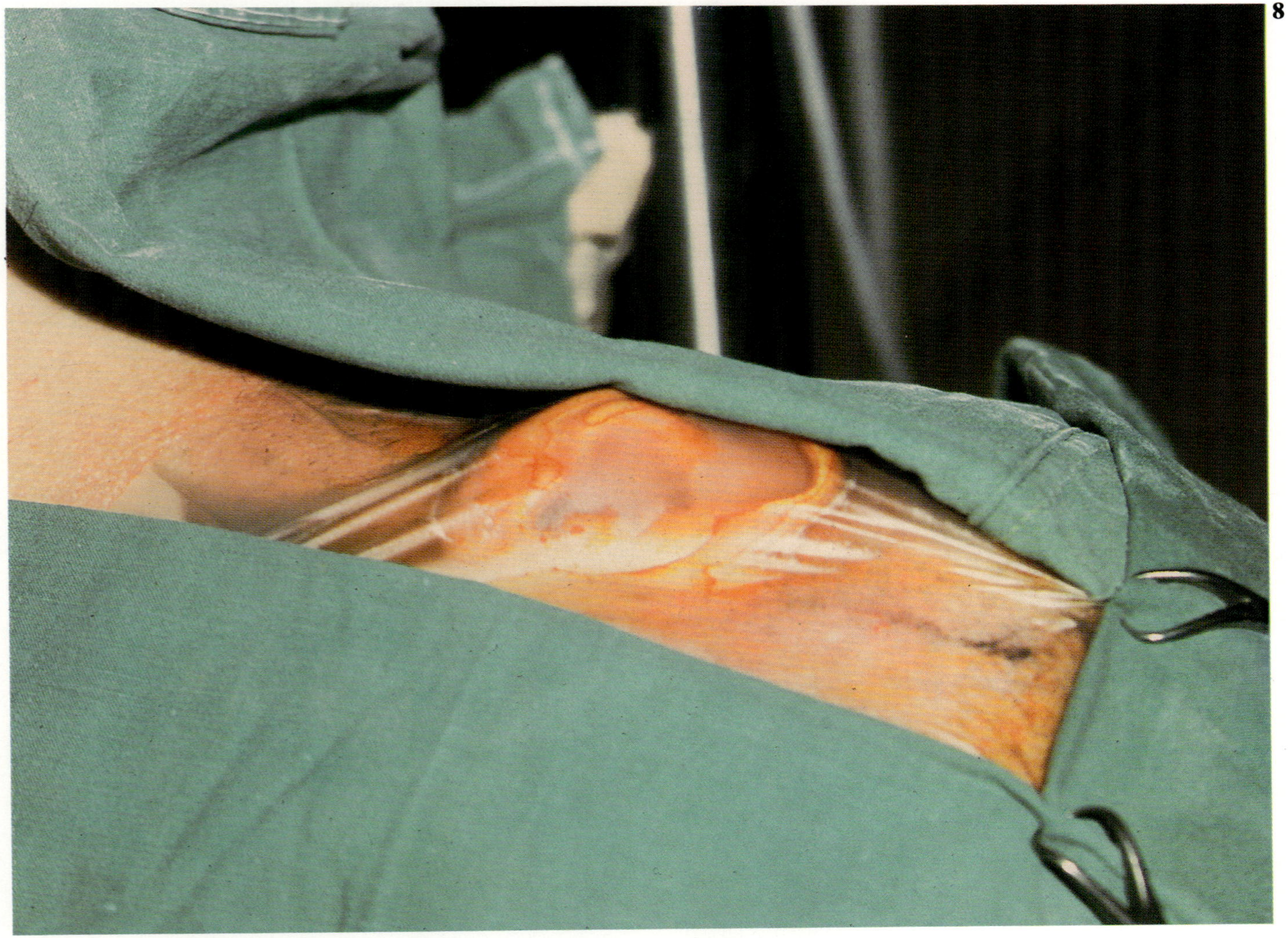

9 A paper towel has been covered by a second layer of green linen towels placed over the shoulder region.

10 A microscope sealing towel is in position, a clip is being applied below the horizontal arm which will later be swung into the field.

11 Sleek is used to stick the upper edge of the microscope towel to the microscope to prevent slipping at a later stage.

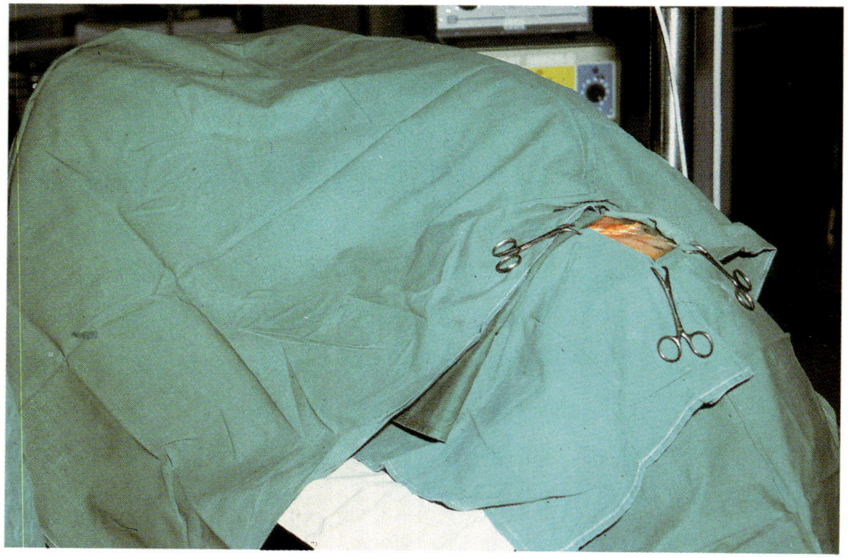
9

10
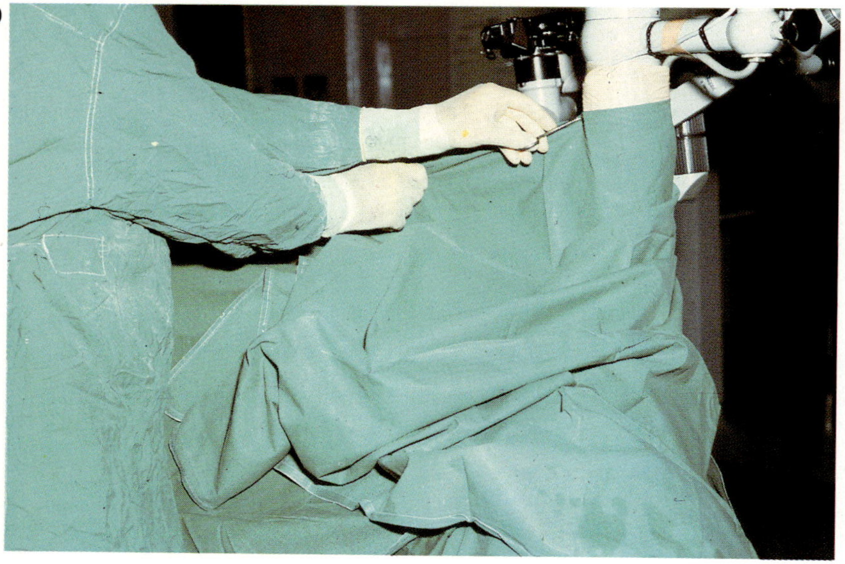

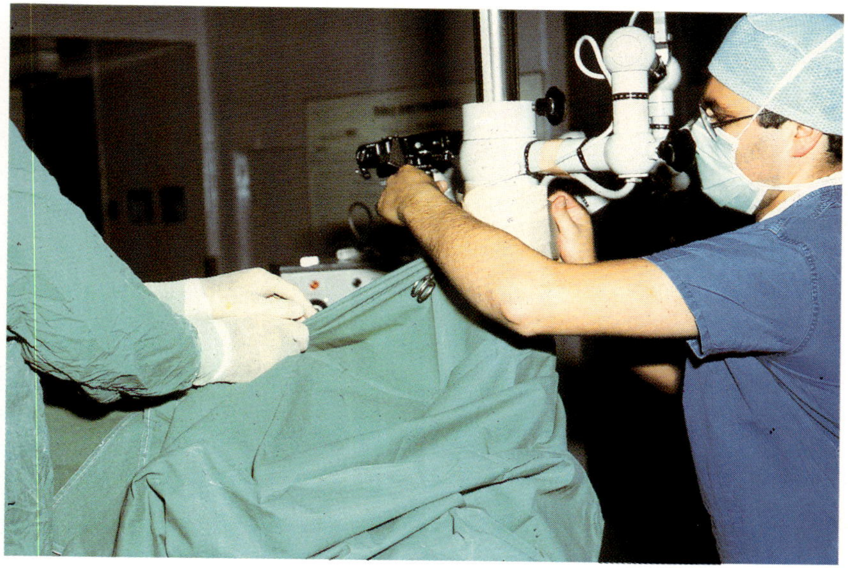
11

12 A thyroid towel covers the full length of the patient. The cranial sited split exposes the operation field. The two cranial clips are being placed outside the final set of towels.

13 Towelling is completed and a bipolar lead and suction apparatus are in position. The blue rubberised mat contains magnets which serve to retain instruments on the irregular surface.

14 The surgeon is in position ready to commence the operation. A ×4 pair of ocular loupes has been donned for dissecting the superficial temporal artery (the working distance of the loupes is approximately 12 to 14 inches).

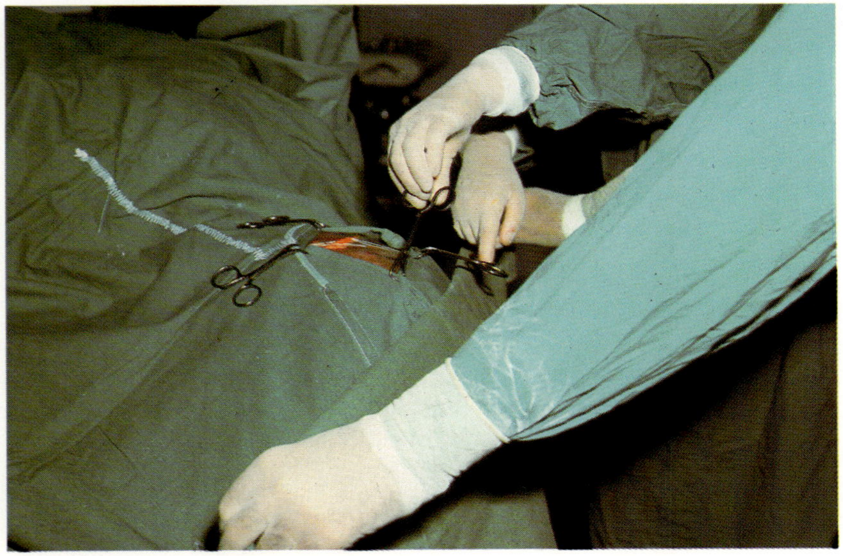

12

13

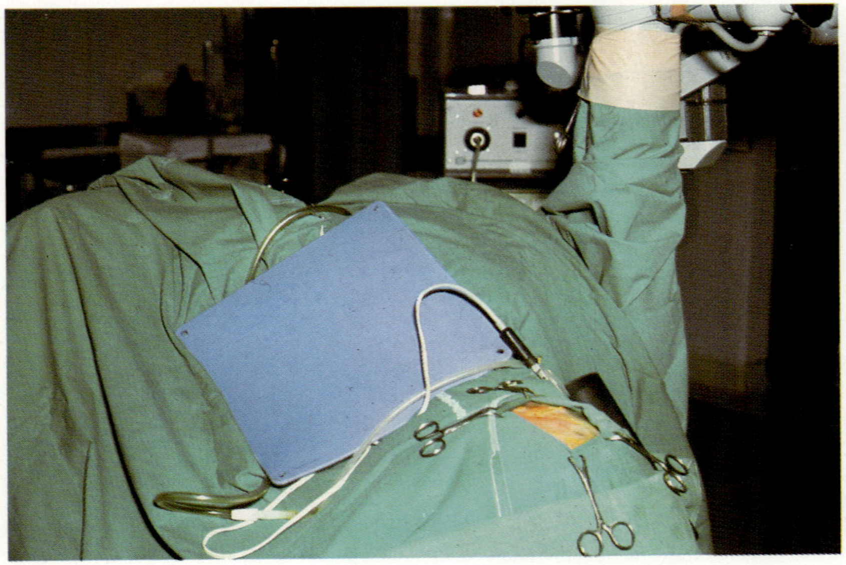

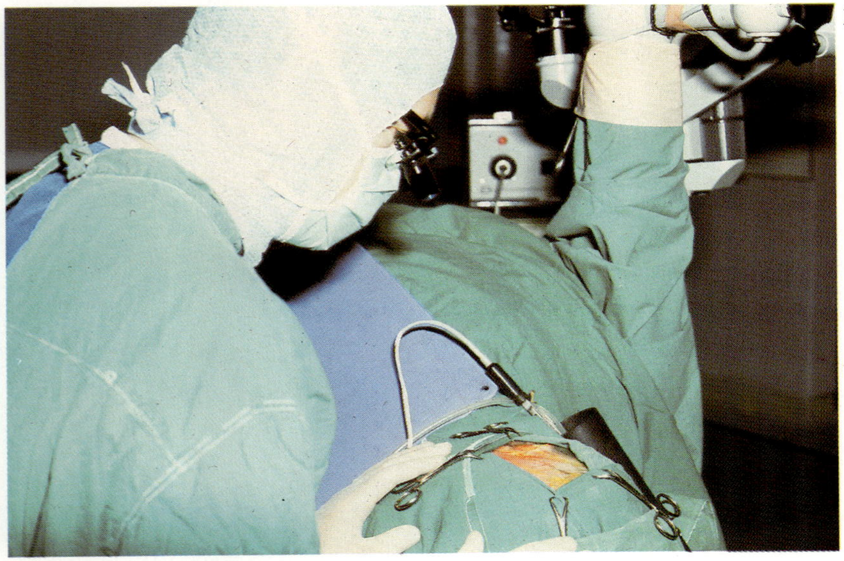

14

Making the incision

15 Initial incision demonstrating the presence of superficial subcuticular vessels which may need haemostasis with a bipolar coagulator. The assistant continually sucks the field dry during the dissection.

16 The subcutaneous plane is developed by blunt dissection with pointed scissors.

17 A mastoid retractor is placed at the subcutaneous level.

15

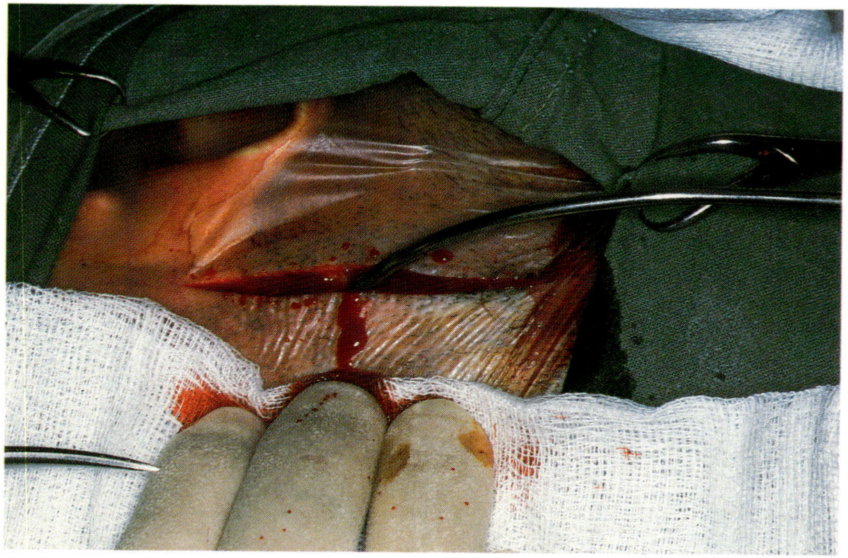

16

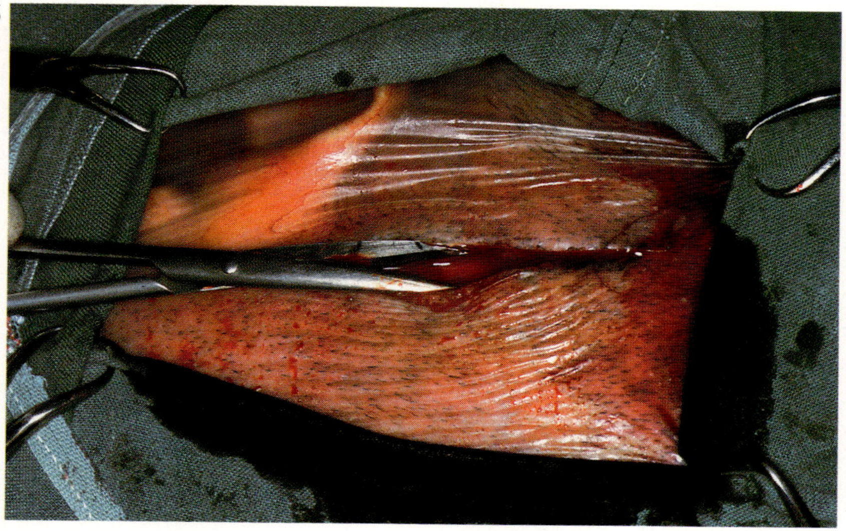

17

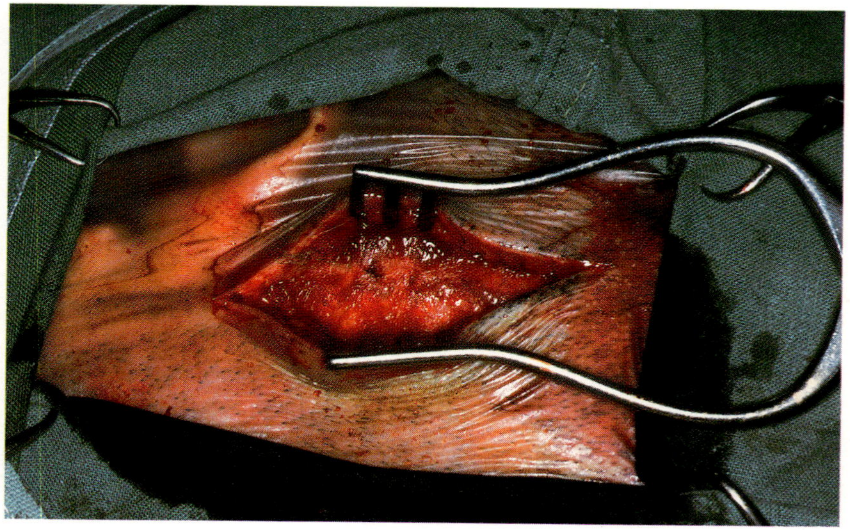

Mobilising superficial tempora artery

18

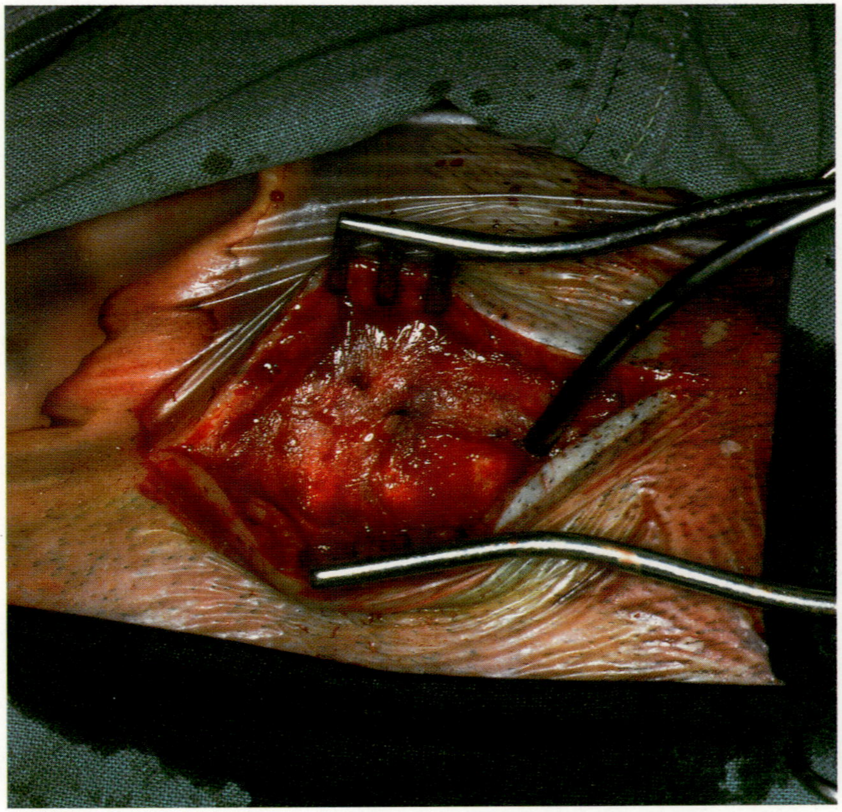

19

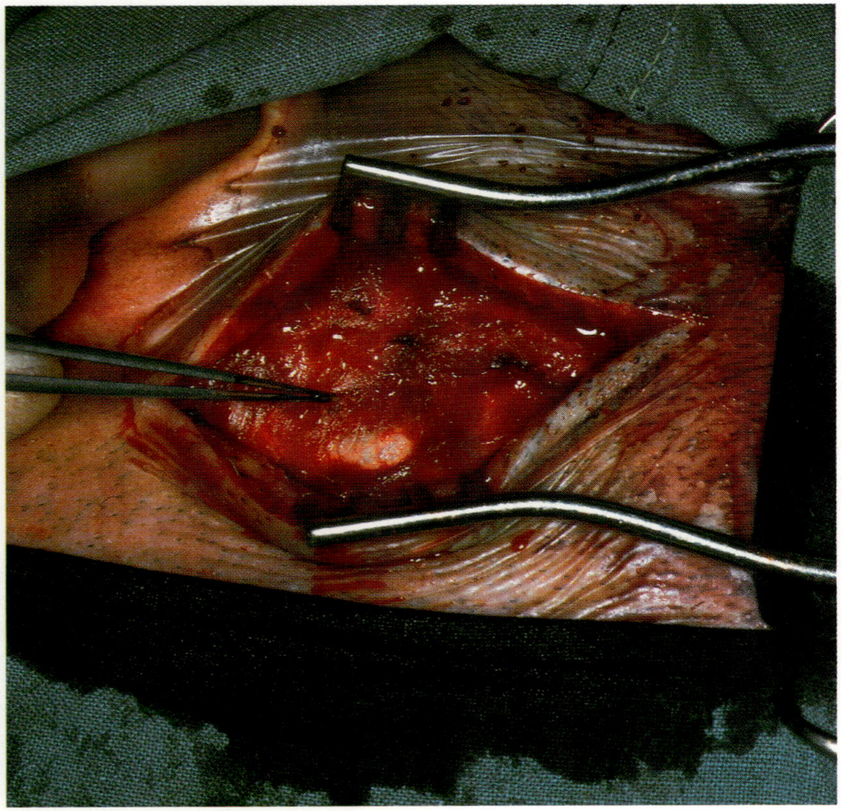

18 Further subcutaneous dissection has taken place and the blades of the retractor are opened more widely. The plane has been deepened anterior to the superficial temporal vessels to the level of the temporalis fascia. The artery can just be seen through the surrounding tissues near the tip of the sucker.

19 Further dissection anterior to the vessels. A bipolar forceps is being used to coagulate the small branches from the artery which can occur anywhere along its length.

20

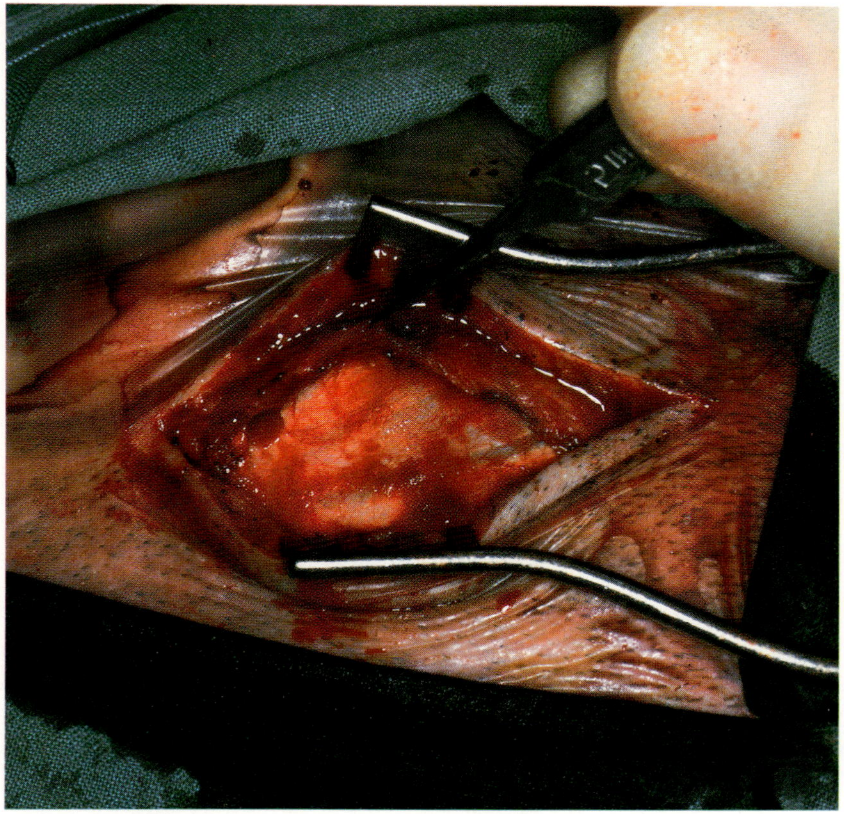

21

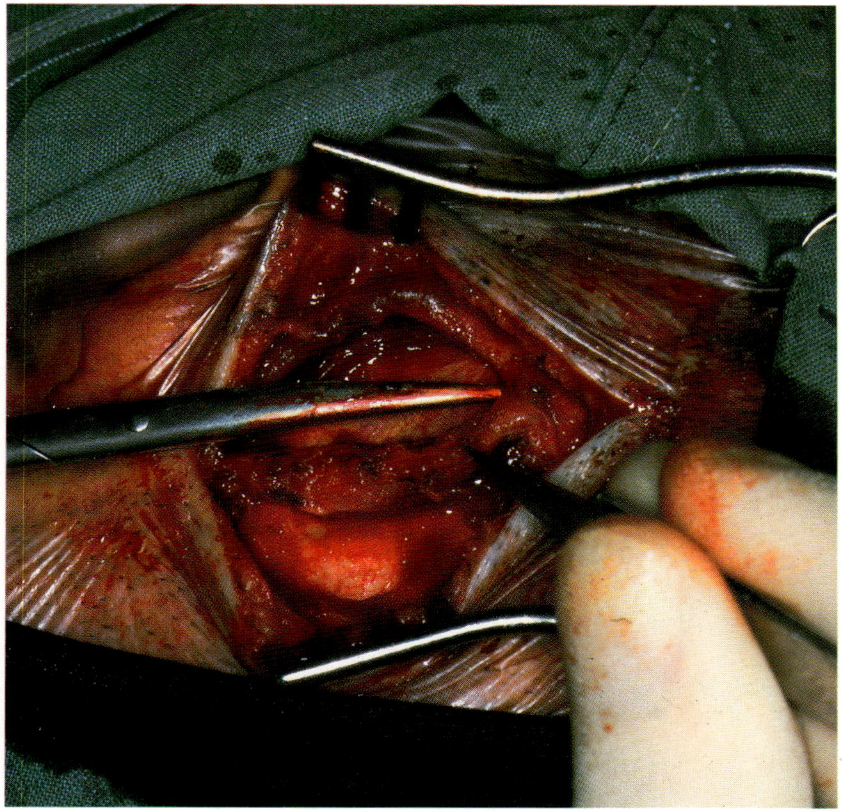

20 The anterior dissection onto the temporalis fascia is now complete and the subcutaneous tissue, containing the superficial temporal vessels, is raised with a watchmaker forceps.

21 The plane of dissection posterior to the superficial temporal artery is being opened. The plane passes between the artery anteriorly and the vein posteriorly; the latter can be seen along the edge of the posterior dissection. Note that the self-retaining retractor has been progressively opened throughout this dissection.

22 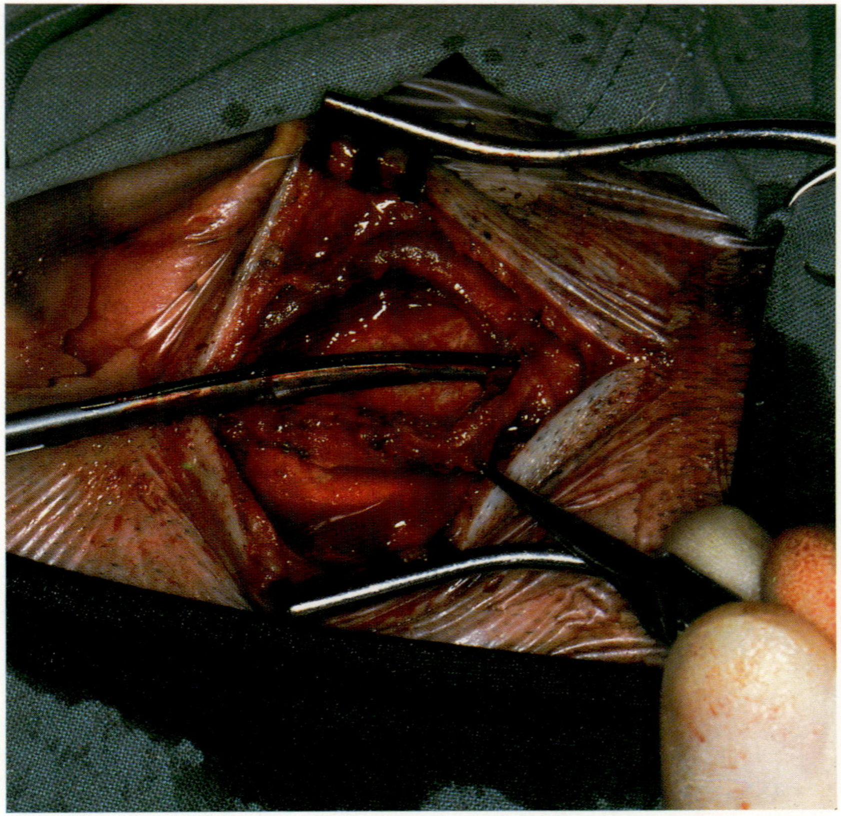

22 Further dissection of the superficial temporal artery pedicle from its surroundings.

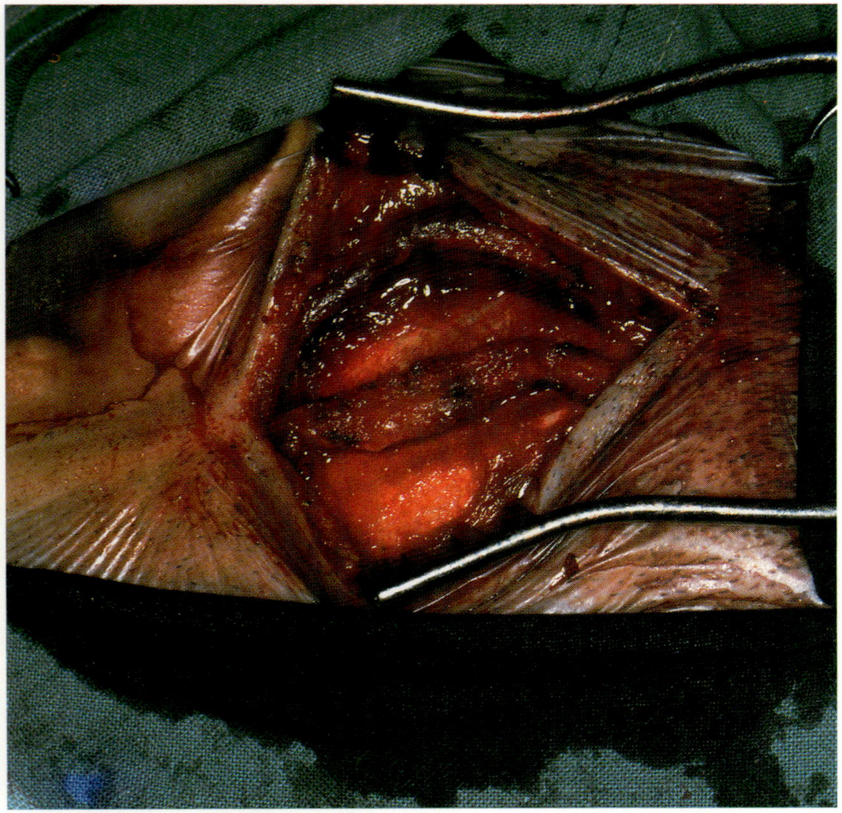 23

23 The dissection of the superficial temporal artery pedicle is complete. Note that the artery is still surrounded by a good deal of local tissue, dissection being kept away from the advential plane to avoid vascular damage.

Division of temporalis fascia

24

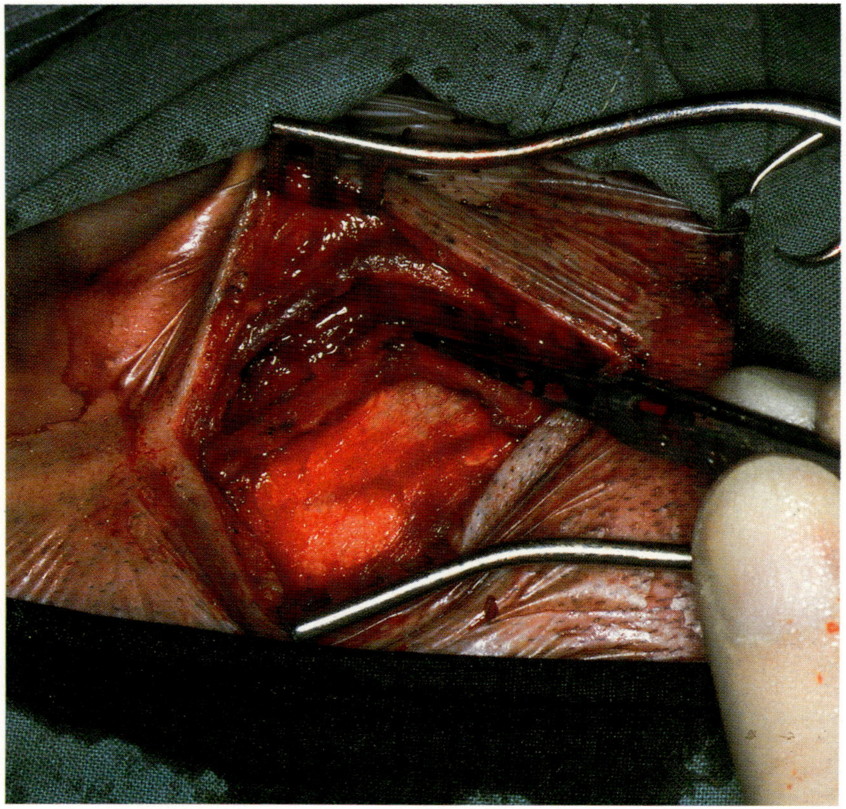

24 The superficial temporal pedicle is lifted to show that the deep clearance is complete.

25

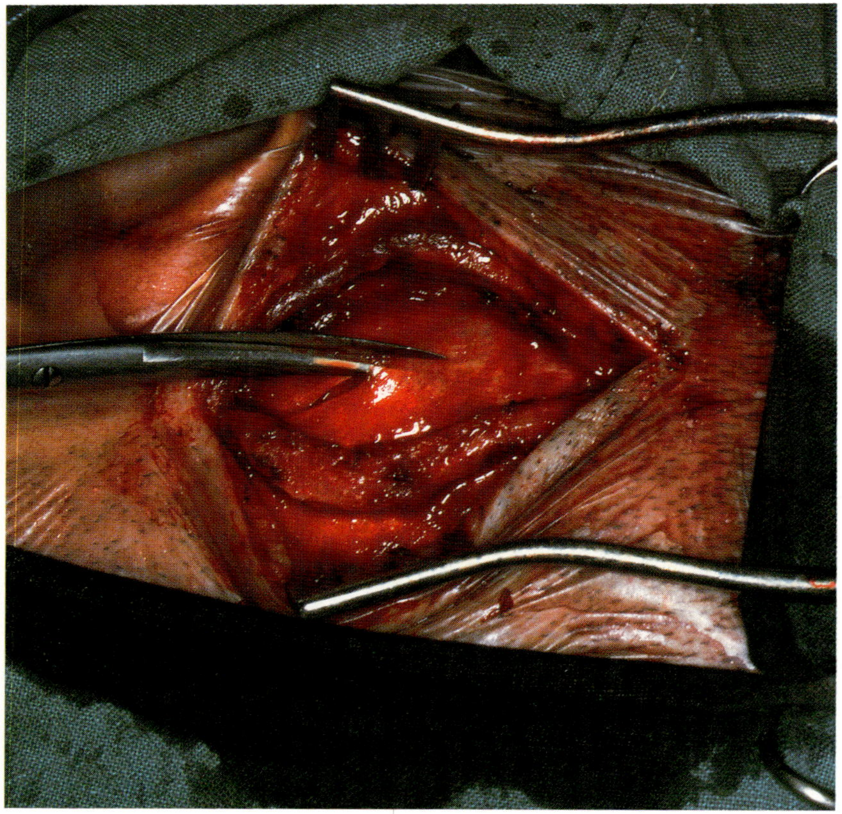

25 The pedicle is placed to one side and the temporalis fascia is being divided in the line of the skin incision.

26

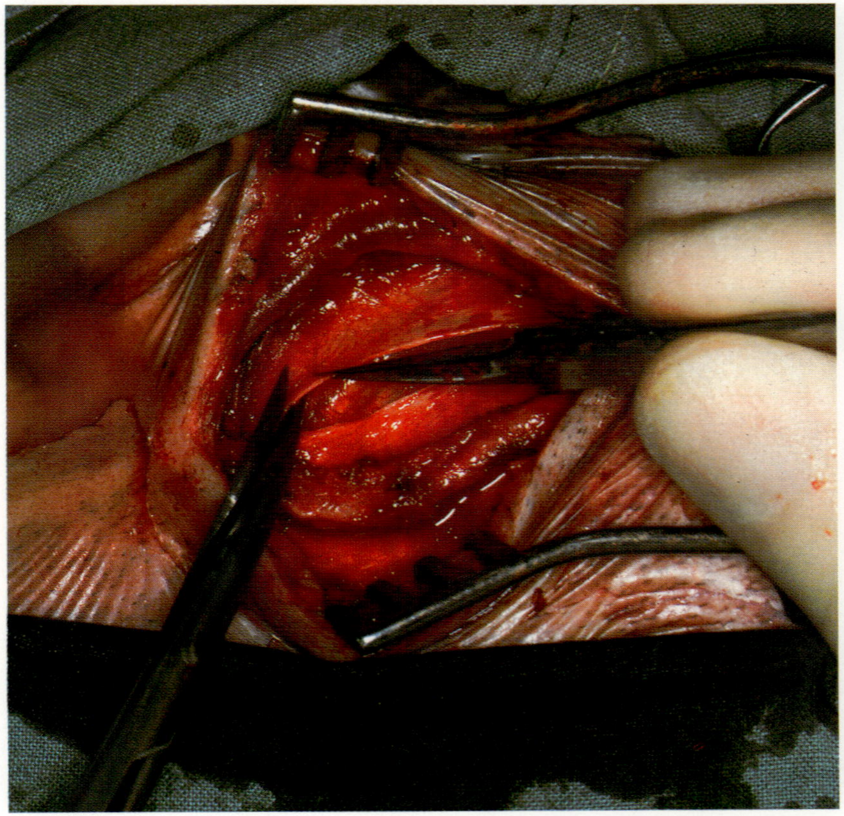

26 The fascia is divided in T fashion to allow subsequent passage of the bypass artery.

27

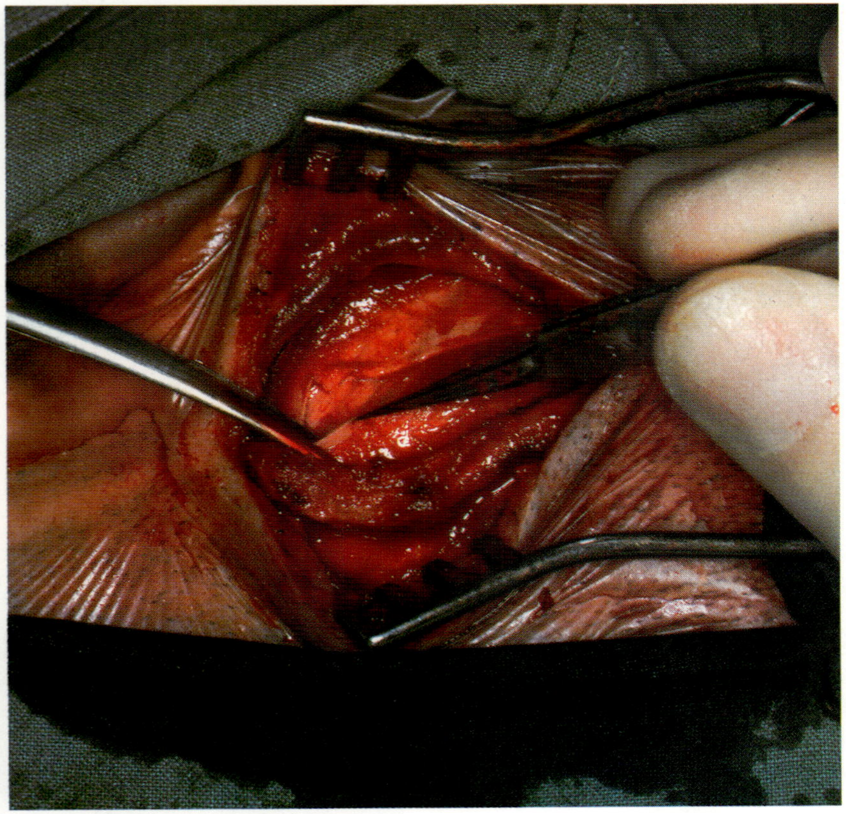

27 The T being extended anteriorly.

28

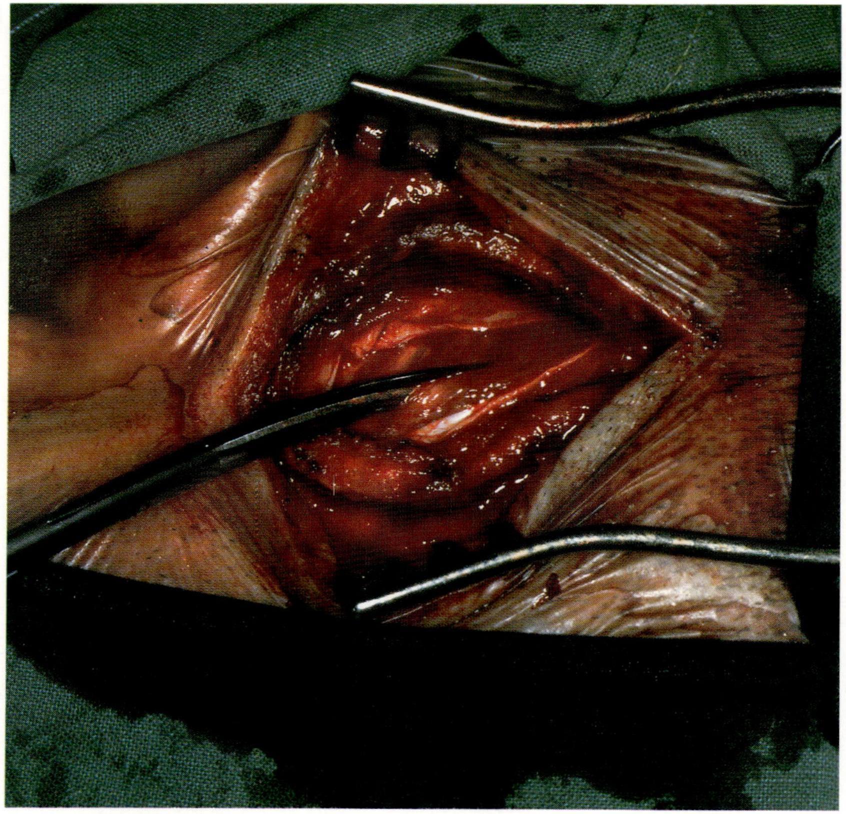

29

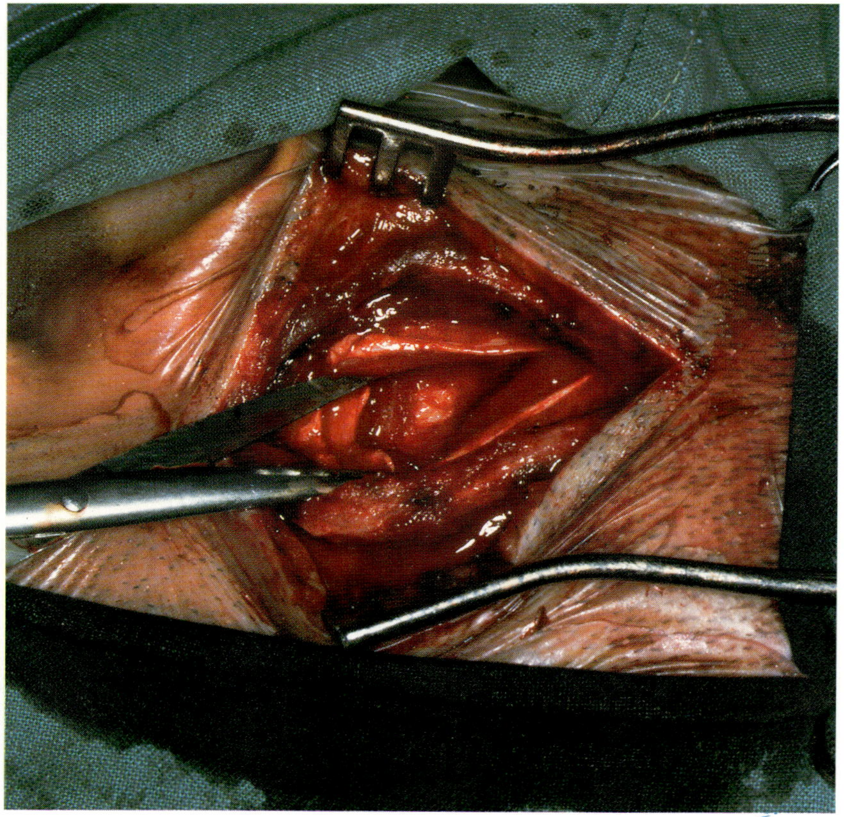

28 A plane of dissection is opened up through the temporalis muscle. This is by both sharp and blunt dissection, muscle fibres crossing the direction of the skin incision being divided, whereas those running along the course of the incision are separated. A number of small vessels passing through the muscle require bipolar coagulation during this dissection.

29 Dissection nearing the skull.

30

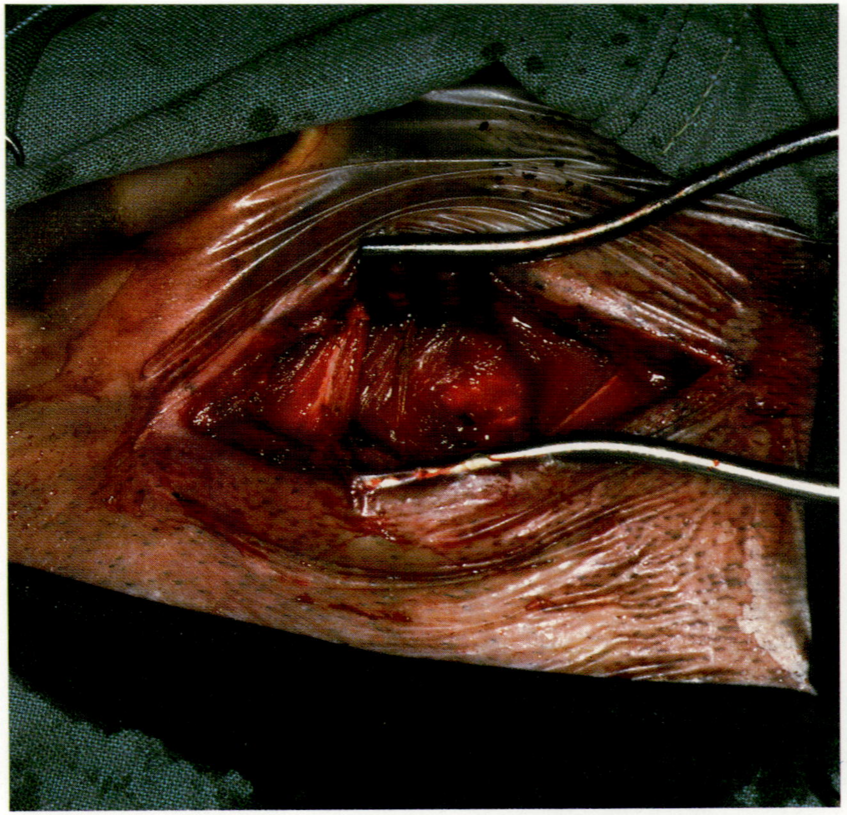

30 The mastoid retractor has been repositioned at a deeper level; it is now separating the anterior and posterior fibres of the temporalis muscle on either side of the dissection.

31

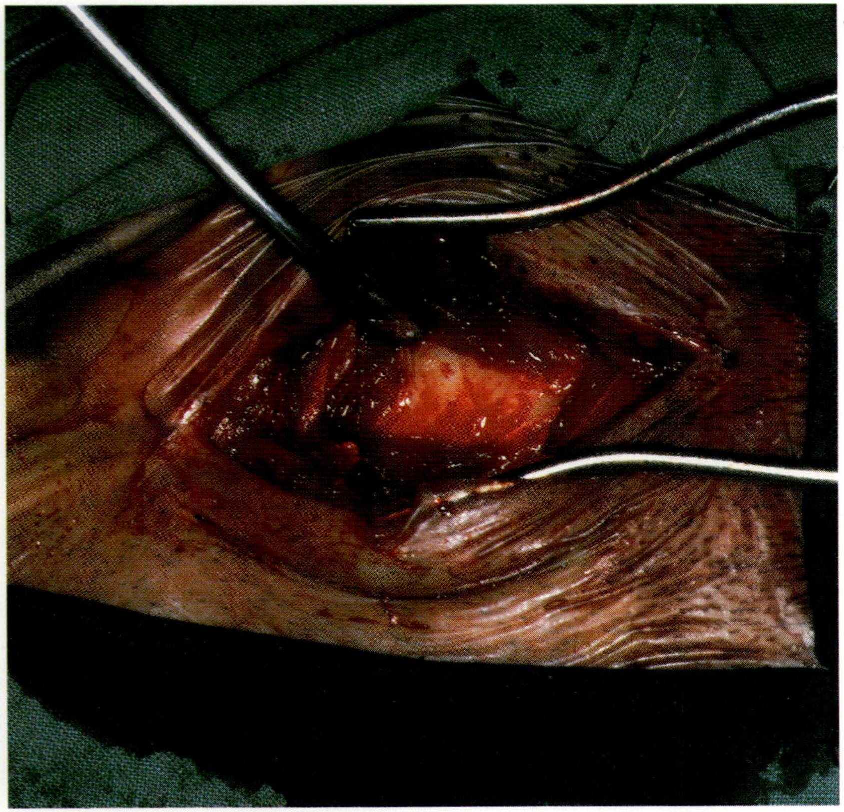

31 The periosteum is scraped away from the exposed bone with an Adson dissector.

Fashioning burr hole

32

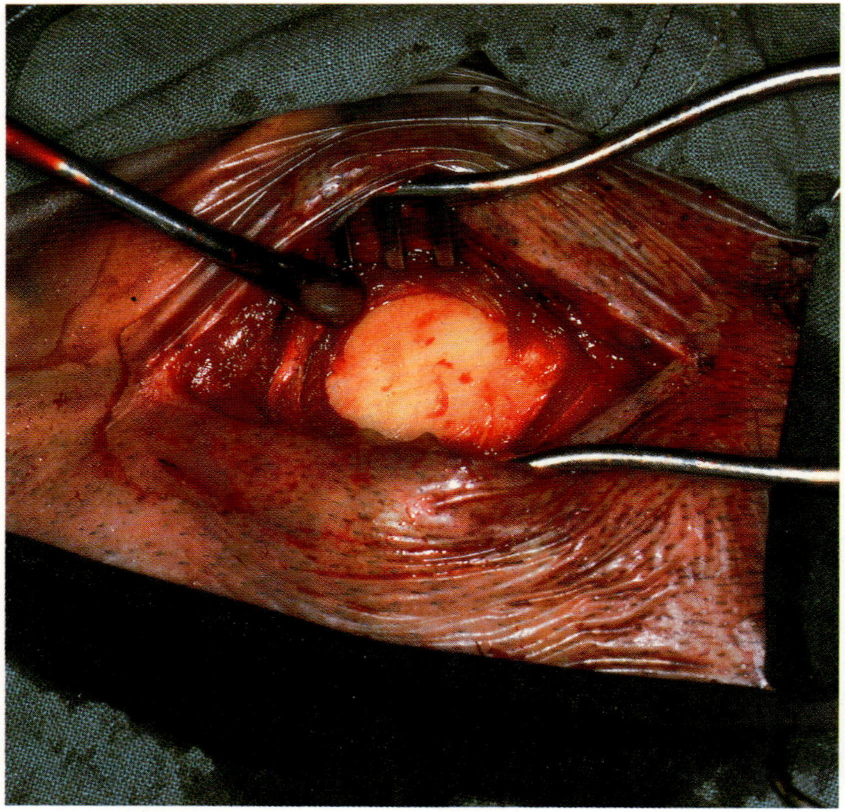

32 Bony exposure complete, ready for the burr hole.

33

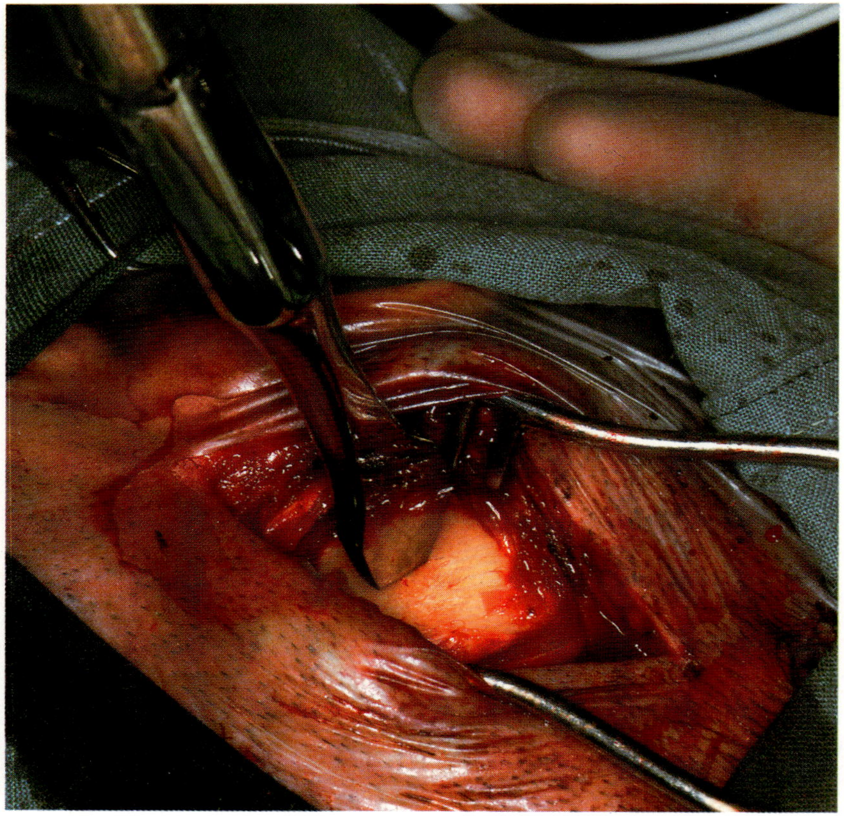

33 Commencement of burr hole. The assistant is steadying the patient's head.

34

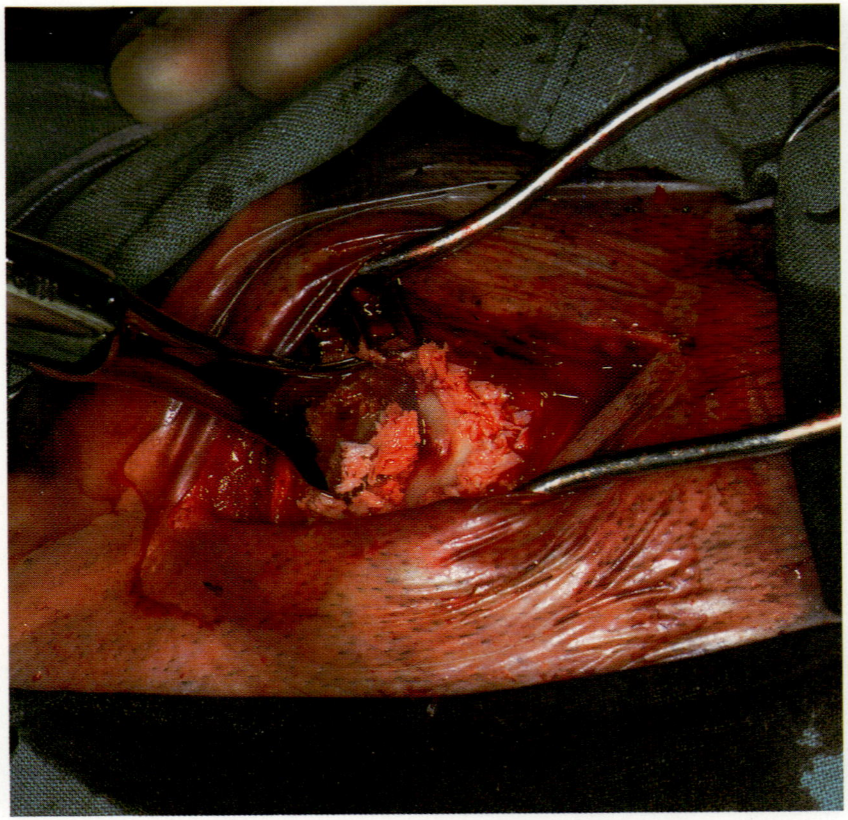

35

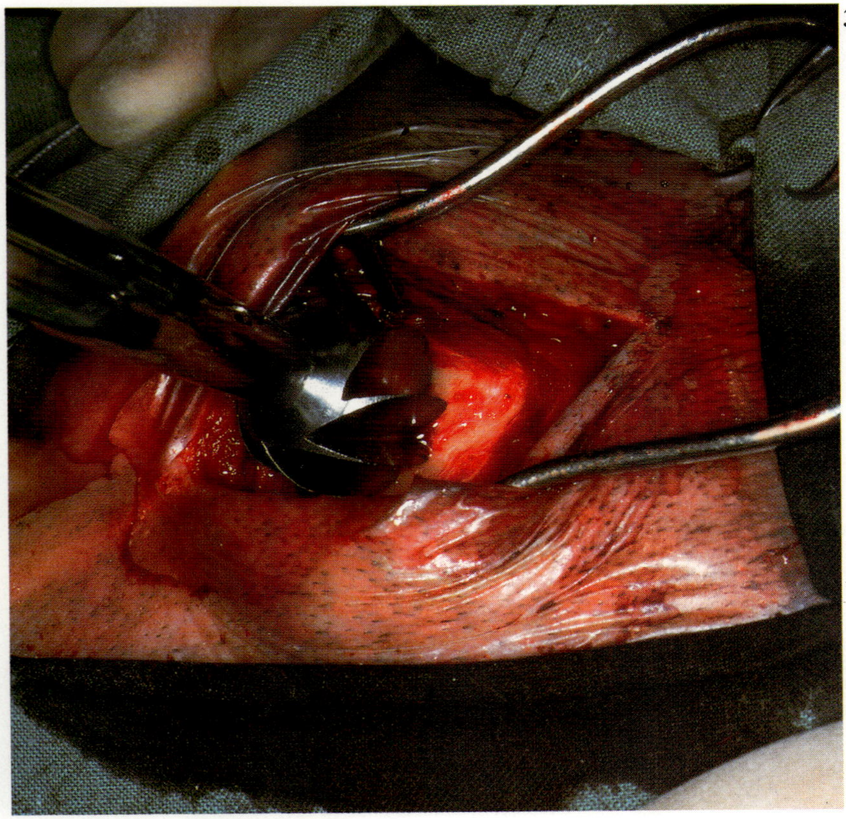

34 Burr hole proceeding. A small amount of saline has been applied to facilitate rotation of the instrument. As the point of the bit reaches the dura, slight unsteadiness is felt on the rotating brace and the bit is replaced with a rose burr. The bone filings are preserved for later replacement.

35 Rose burr in position. This is approximately 1 cm in diameter.

Dural incision

36

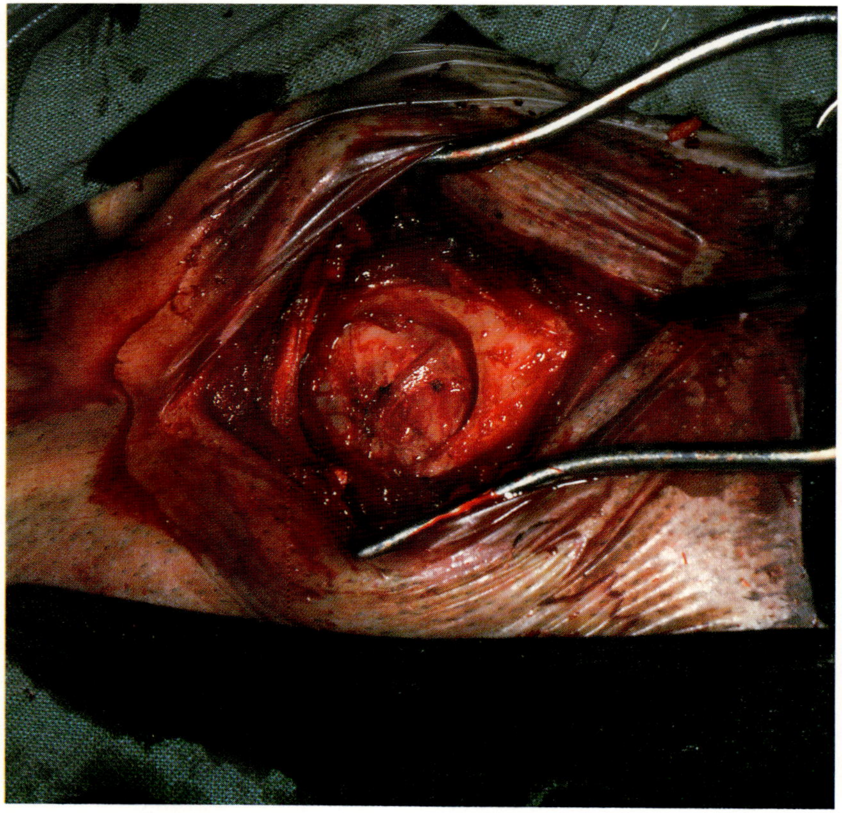

37

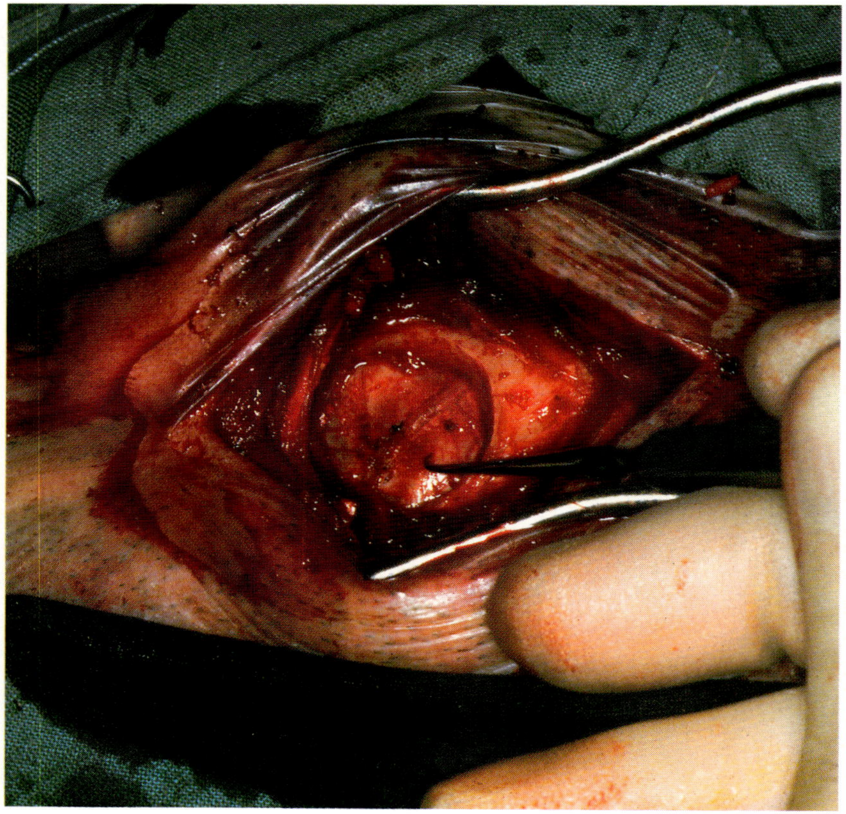

36 Completed burr hole. Wax is sometimes needed to control bleeding from the bony edge or small vessels closely applied to it. The middle meningeal artery is seen crossing the centre of the burr hole with its dural coverings.

37 A dural hook is applied to one side of the middle meningeal artery ready for incision parallel to the vessel using a pointed scalpel blade.

38

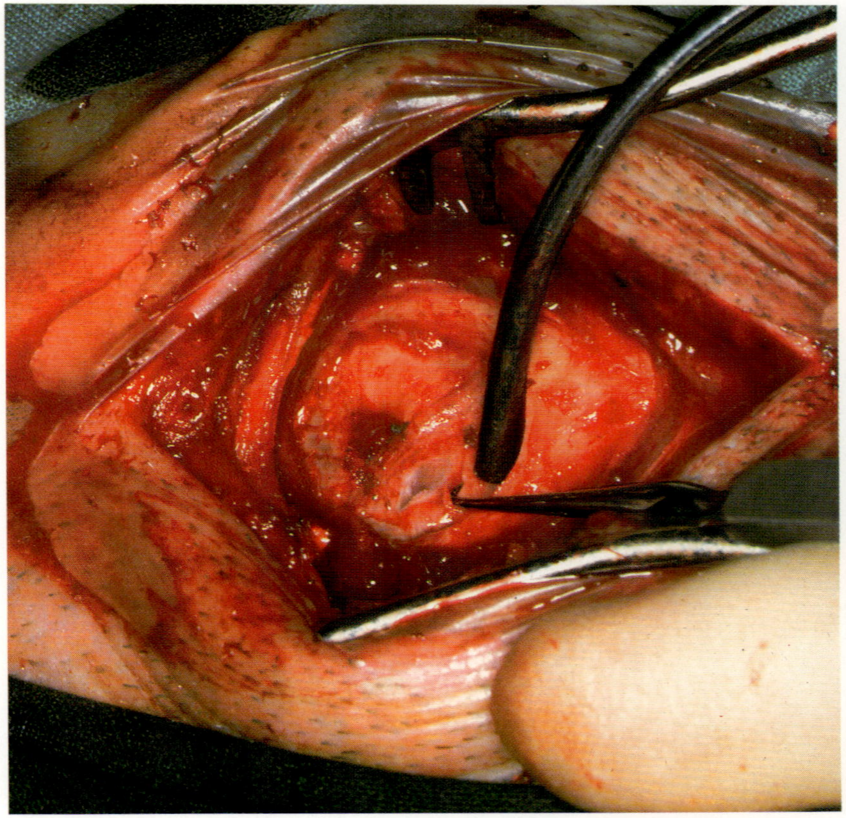

39

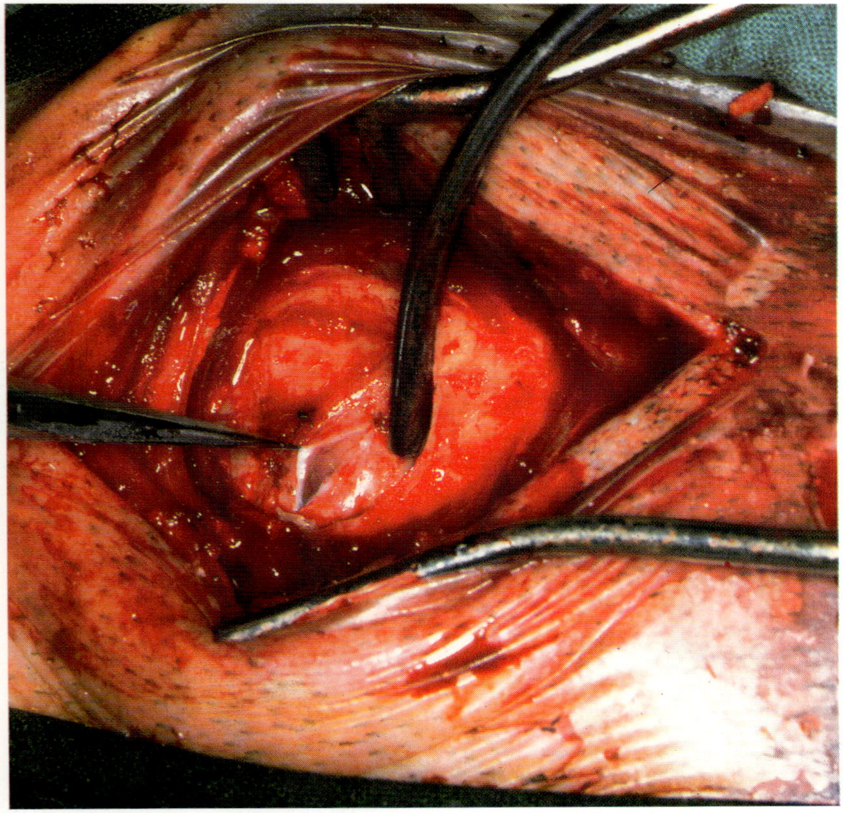

38 The dural incision has been started. The underlying transparent arachnoid is still intact and the cortex can be seen.

39 Watchmaker forceps raising an edge of the divided duramater; an underlying artery of approximately 1 mm in diameter is present and suitable for anastomosis. If a satisfactory vessel is not immediately located, the dura is divided in stellate fashion and the bone nibbled away in the line of the lateral sulcus. Bony extension of the burr hole is required in about a third of patients.

40 After identification of a satisfactory cortical vessel further dural incision can be left for dissection under the microscope. A pattie is placed in the bony defect and the mastoid retractor temporarily removed. This manoeuvre allows freeing of the superficial temporal pedicle which has been displaced beneath one jaw of the retractor during the burr hole and dural dissection. The retractor is replaced, retracting the temporalis muscle and leaving the superficial temporal artery pedicle across the middle of the field.

At this stage the surgeon changes over to the operating microscope for the final dissection of the scalp artery, further dural incision and fashioning of the anastomosis. The ocular loupes are removed and the instrument trolleys moved from close proximity to the operative field while the microscope, on its horizontal arm, is brought over the pre-set site; this usually corresponds to the burr hole. If the burr hole has been extended to locate a satisfactory cortical vessel, the microscope may also require slight adjustment of its position. Sterile black caps can be placed over the main two controls on the body of the microscope allowing the surgeon to control this movement; some locking devices will have to be temporarily released during this repositioning.

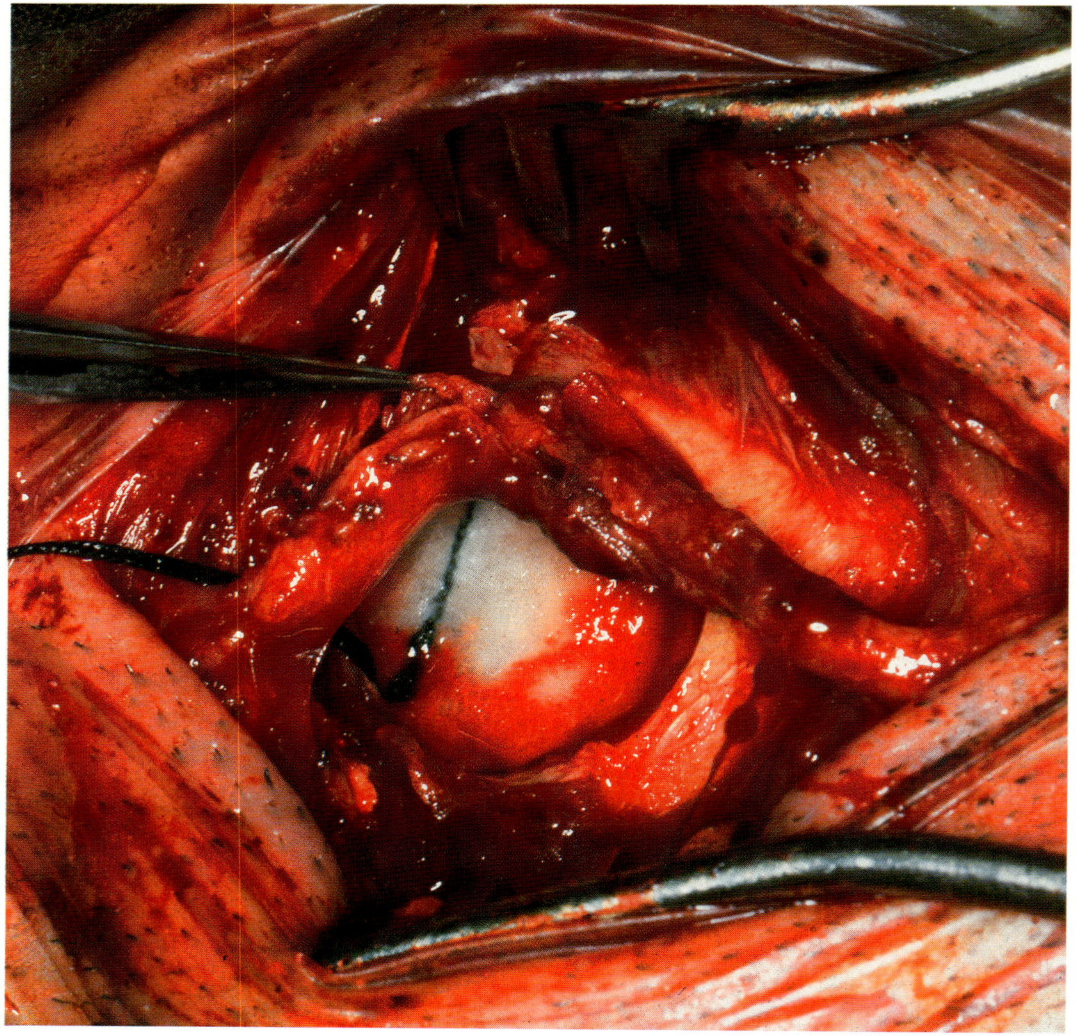

40

Mobilising cortical artery

41 View of the operating field through the operating microscope. The dural incision has been enlarged and the dura retracted back to the inferior left side of the picture. A watchmaker forceps is applied to the arachnoid. The cortical artery to be used for anastomosis is seen through this transparent layer. A vein is present and the underlying sulcus is probably the lateral sulcus.

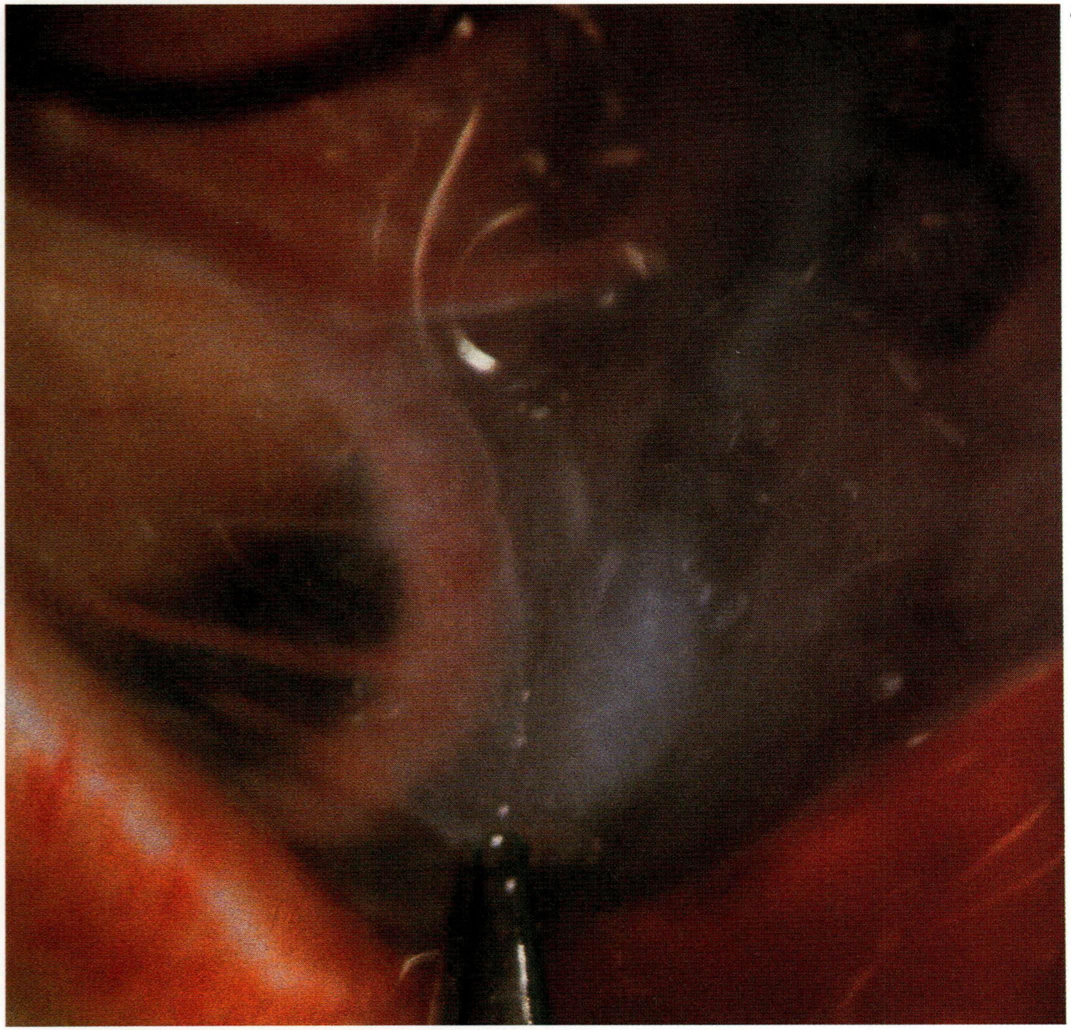

41

42 A second watchmaker forceps is applied to the arachnoid which is being torn gently. Tearing is usually easier than sharp division of the arachnoid, but it must always be undertaken under direct vision so that any minute branches adherent to it can be seen and carefully avoided.

42

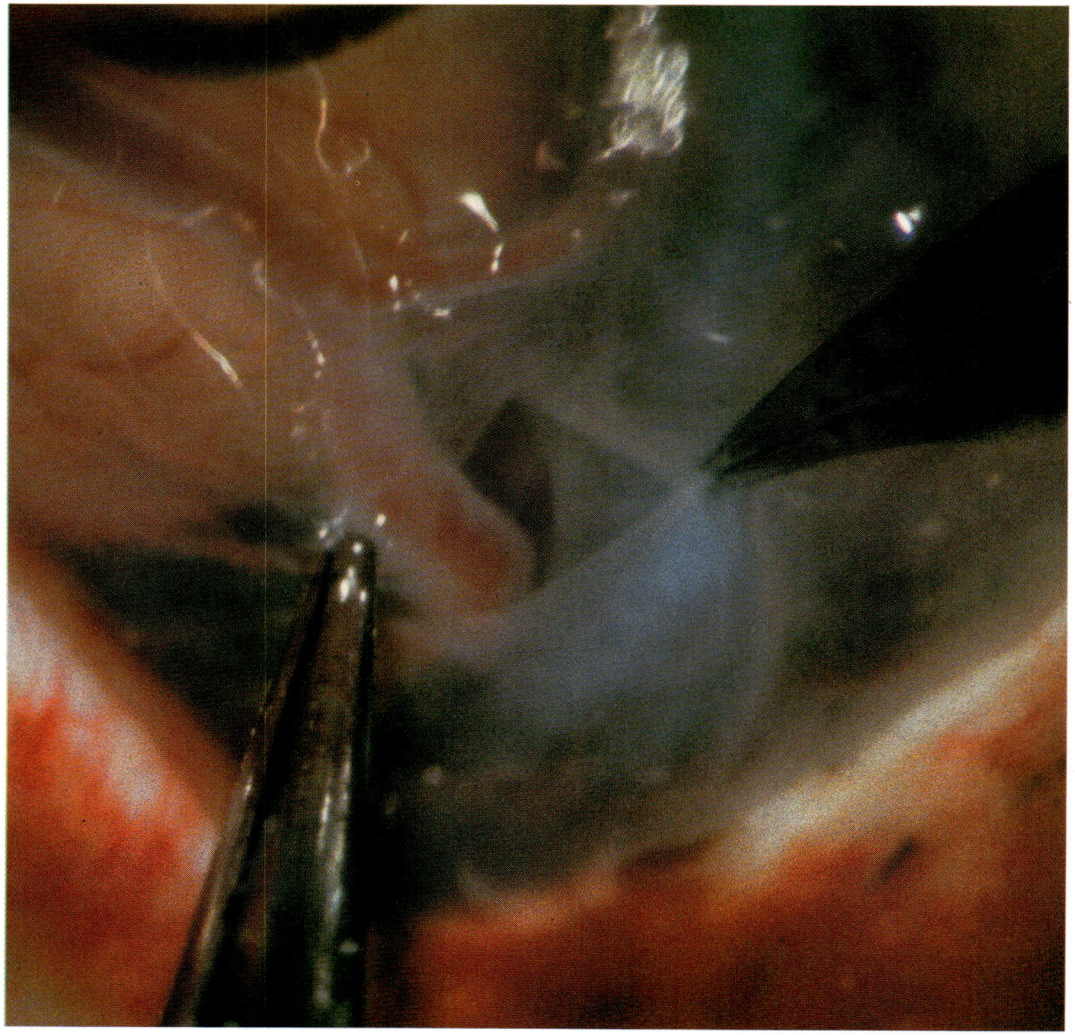

43 **Tear of arachnoid proceeding.**

43

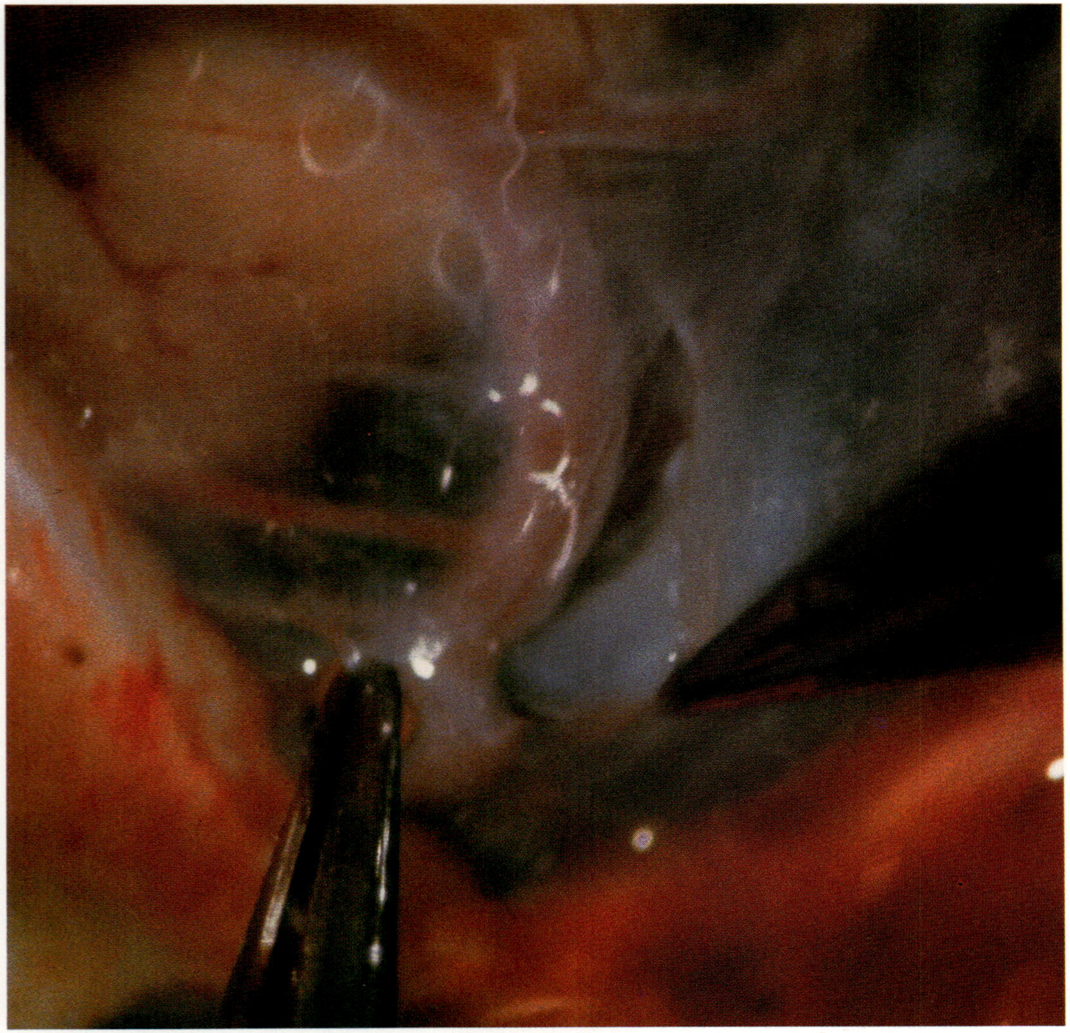

44 The arachnoid has been cleared from the major part of the cortical artery. The vein has been left undisturbed.

44

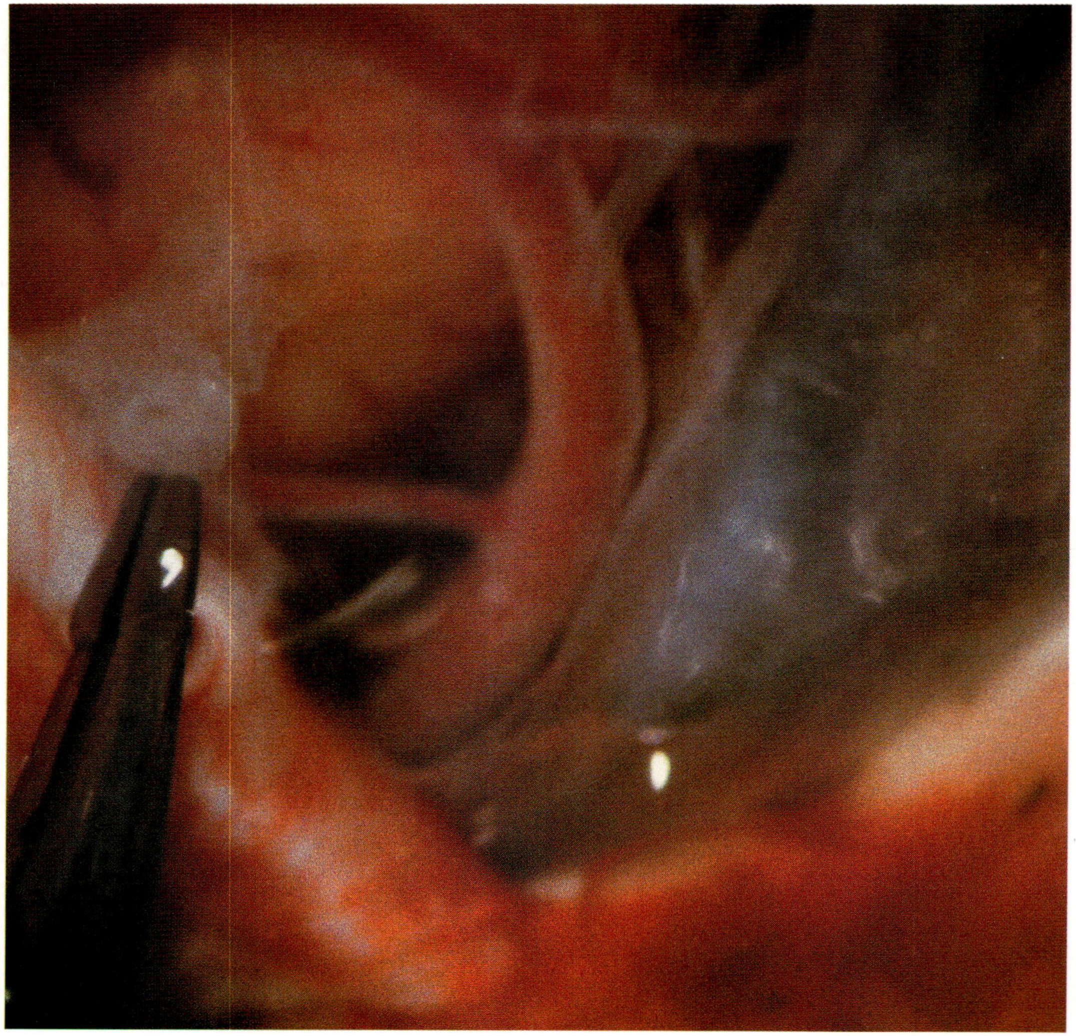

45 Removal of a few more fragments of arachnoid exposing over a 1 cm length of the cortical branch of the middle cerebral artery.

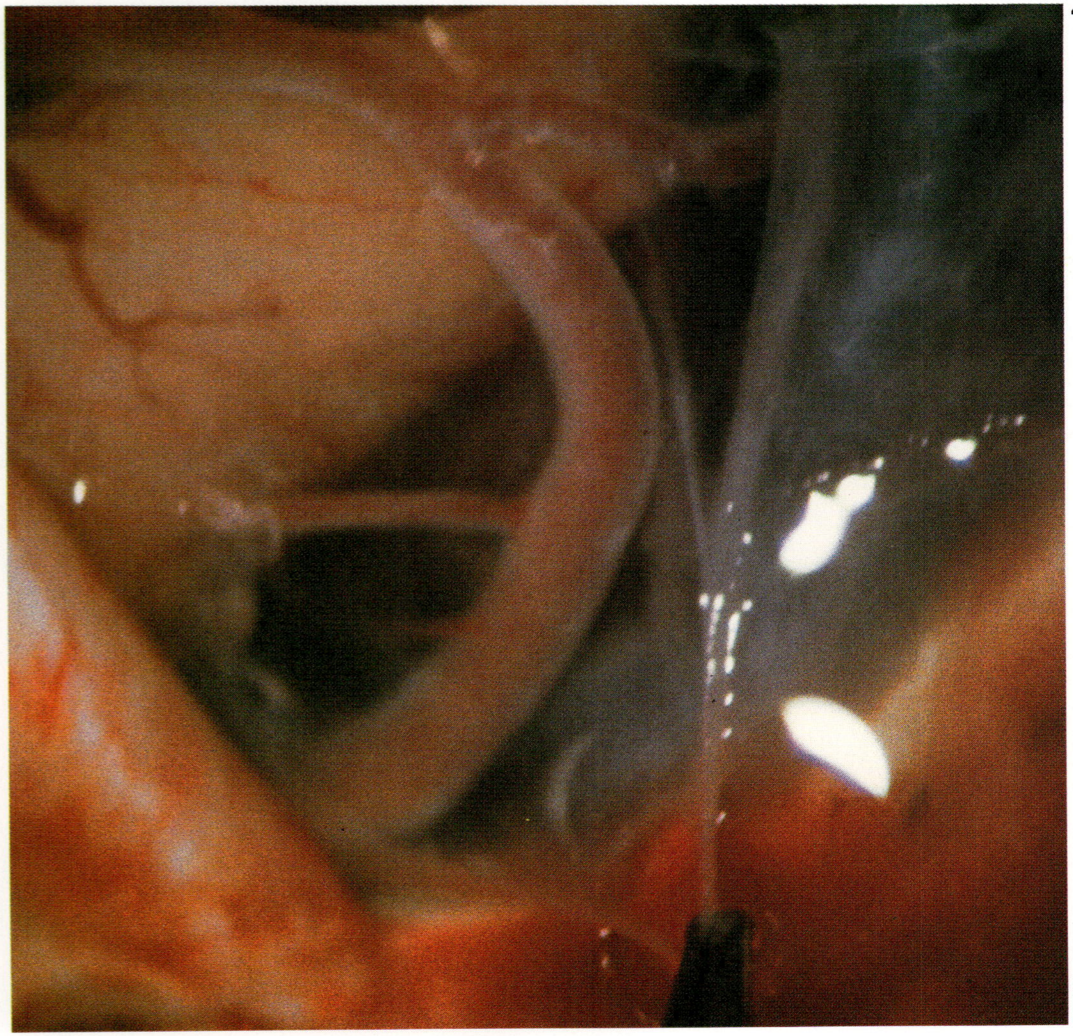
45

Application of clips

46 Application of the first microvascular clip. The cortical artery is being raised with a watchmaker forceps which has been applied to the adventitia, care being taken to avoid damage to the wall of the vessel. The clip is including a small branch in its jaws; this could otherwise back-bleed and add difficulty to the subsequent anastomosis.

46

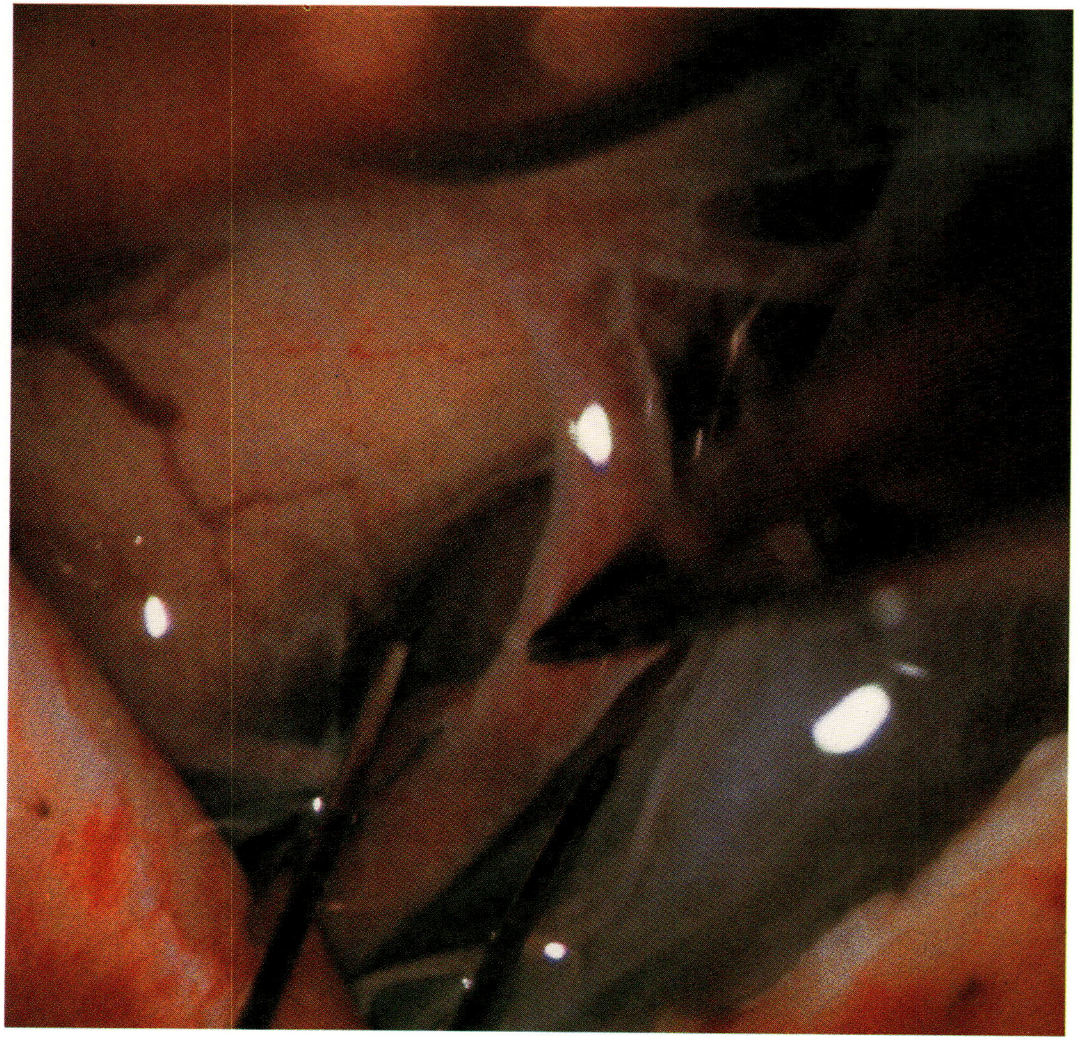

47 Clip in position. Be sure that the locking device on the clip applicator is released before attempting to take the applicator away from the operating field. If it is still attached to the clip at this time, it may cause irredeemable tearing of the cortical vessel.

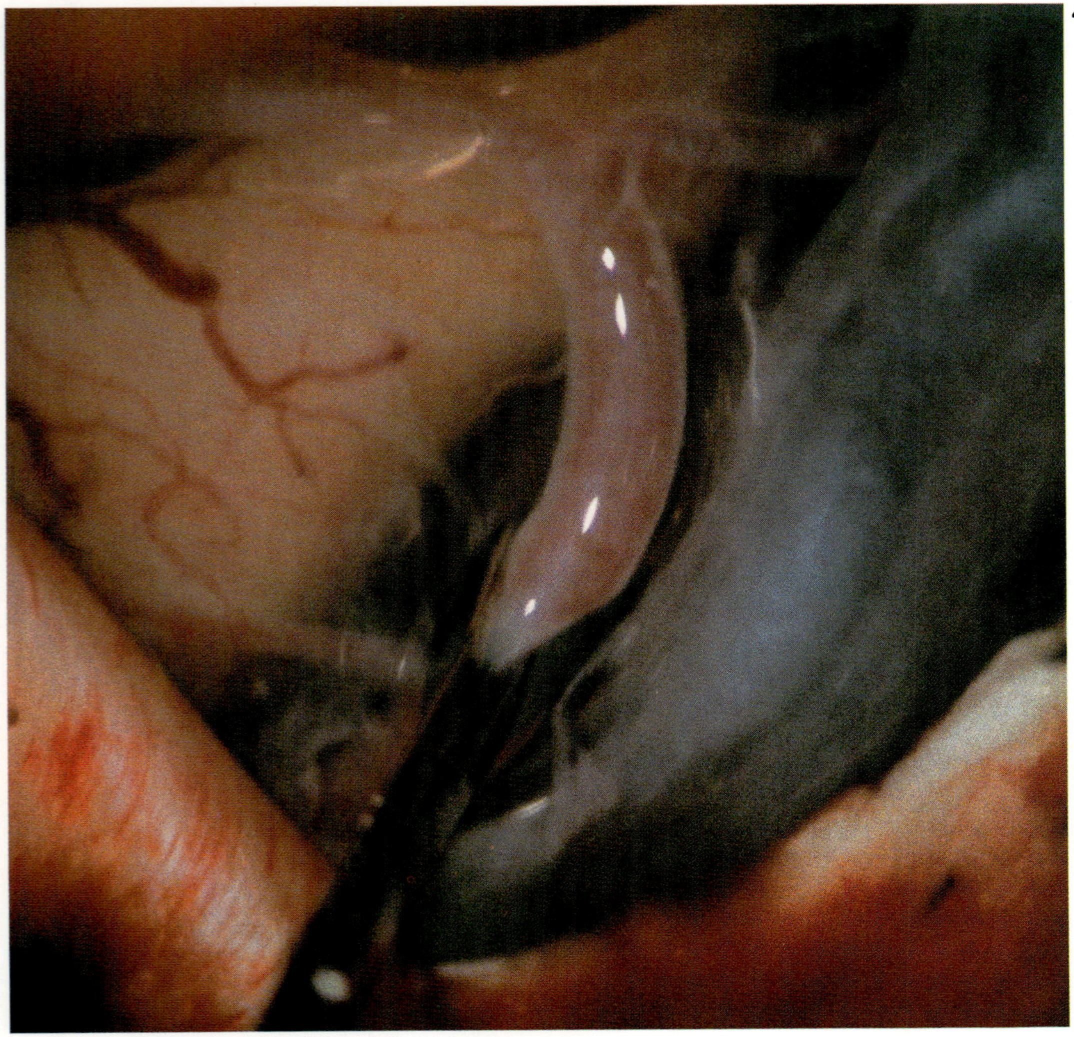
47

48 Application of the second microvascular clip. The forceps' hold on the artery includes a little media on this occasion, because the operator wanted to apply more traction to ensure that the clip was placed near the next branch, thus ensuring as much length of straight unbranched artery as possible for anastomosis. The hold, however, has been applied over the area of the artery which will subsequently be excised.

48

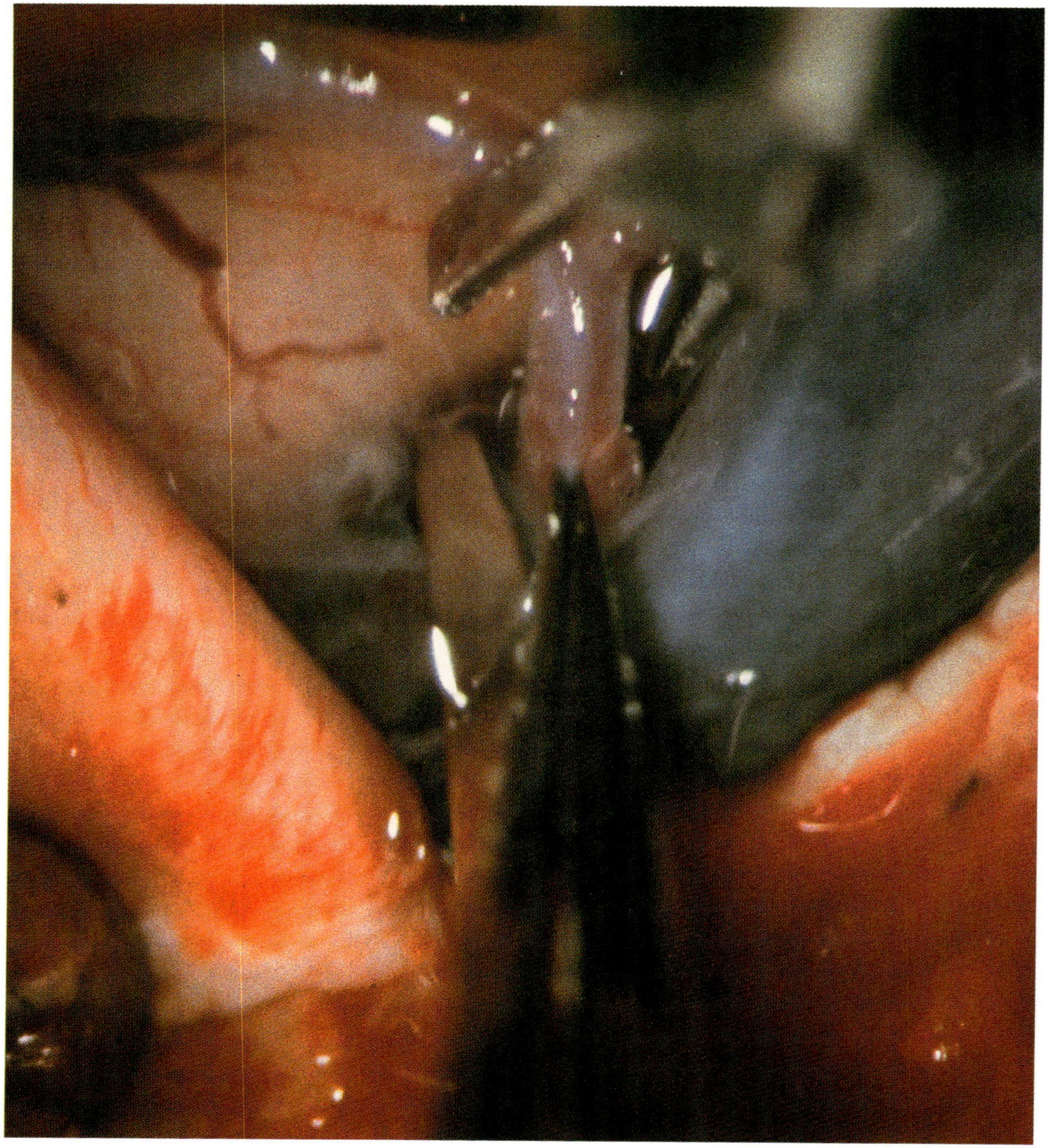

49

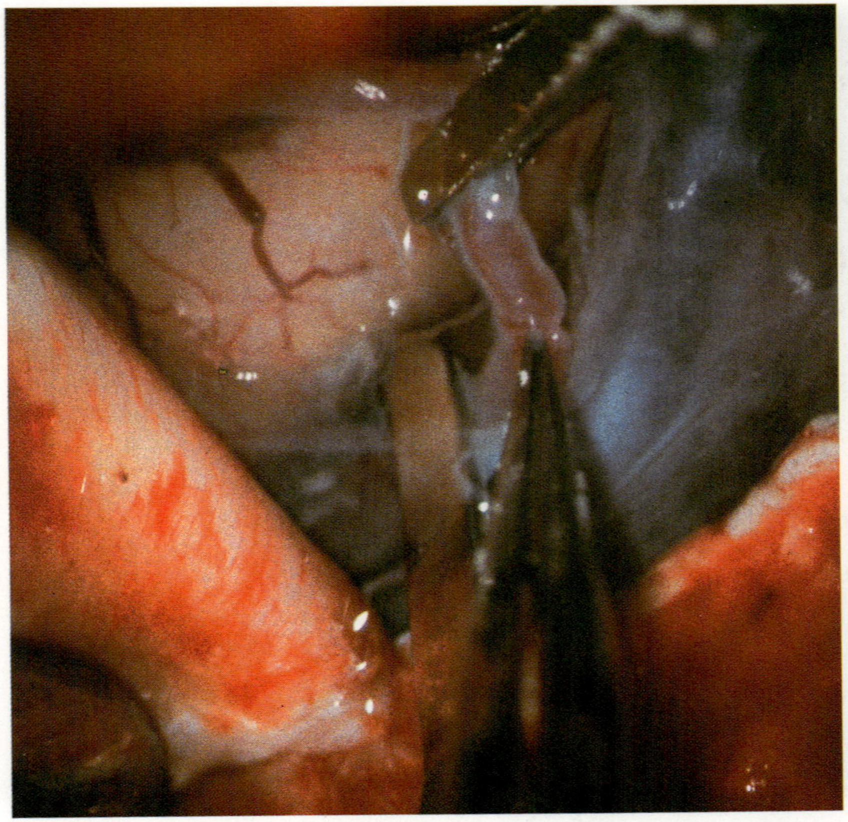

49 **The second clip is in position, the artery is held at the same point of media.**

50

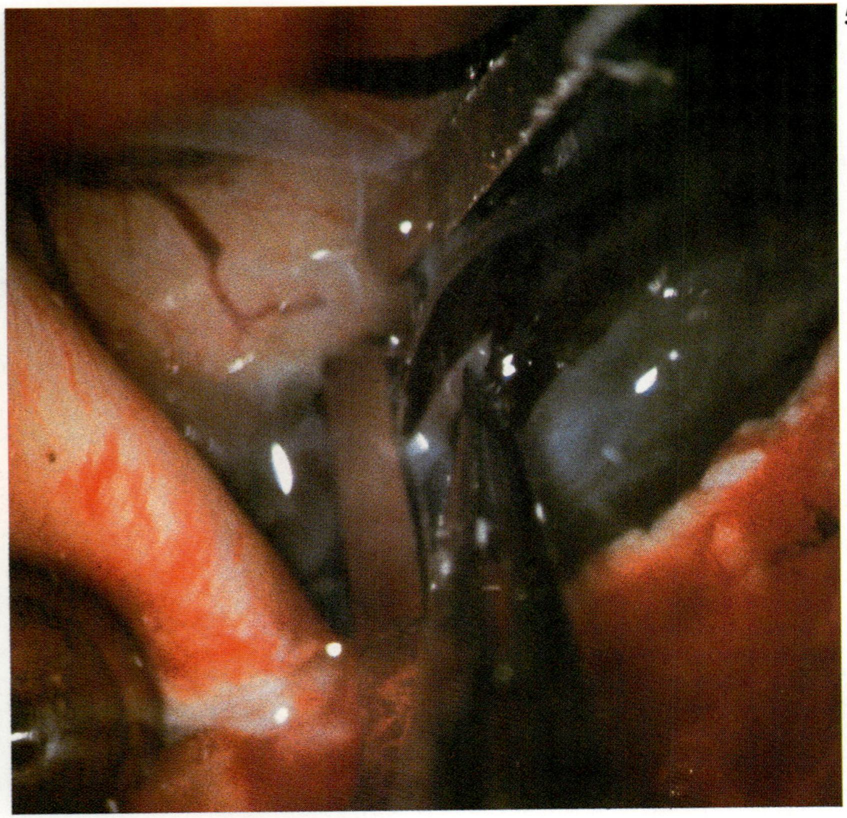

50 **The watchmaker hold is still applied and a segment of the anterior surface of the vessel is being excised** as an ellipse with a curved micro-vascular scissors.

Fashioning superficial temporal artery

51

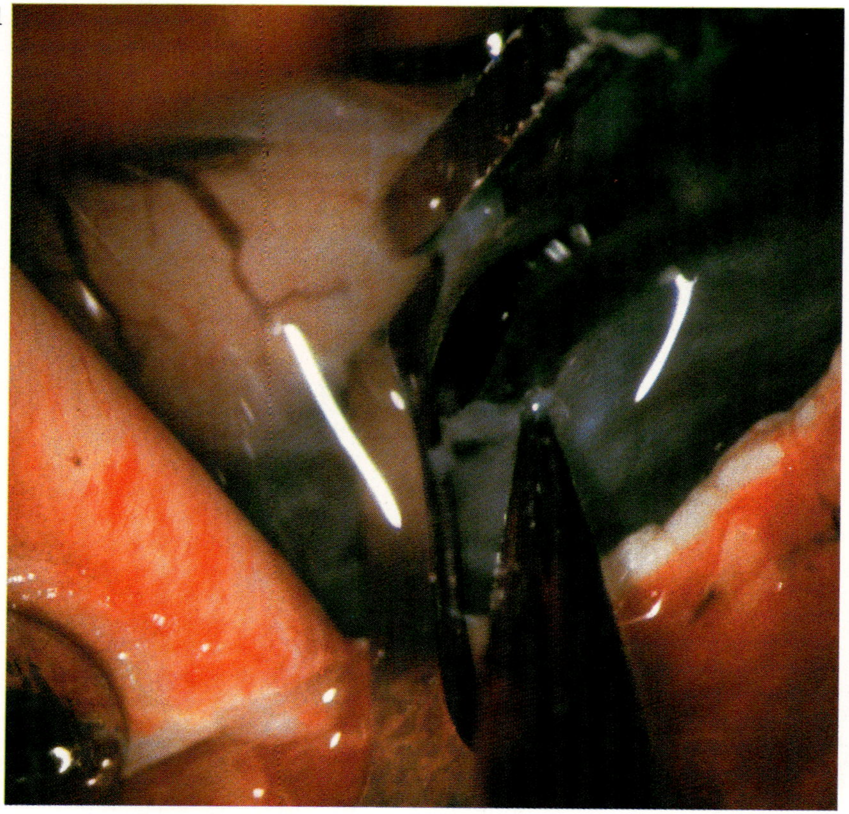

51 A later stage in the removal of the ellipse of cortical vessel.

52

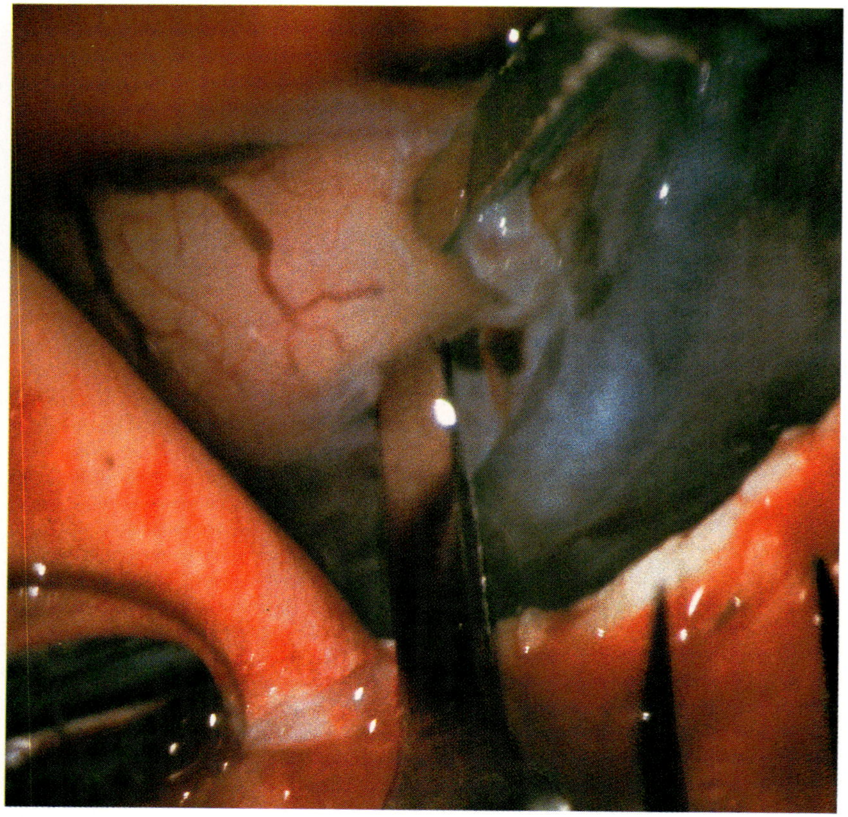

52 Removal of ellipse is complete and residual blood is seen in the clamped segment of cortical artery.

53

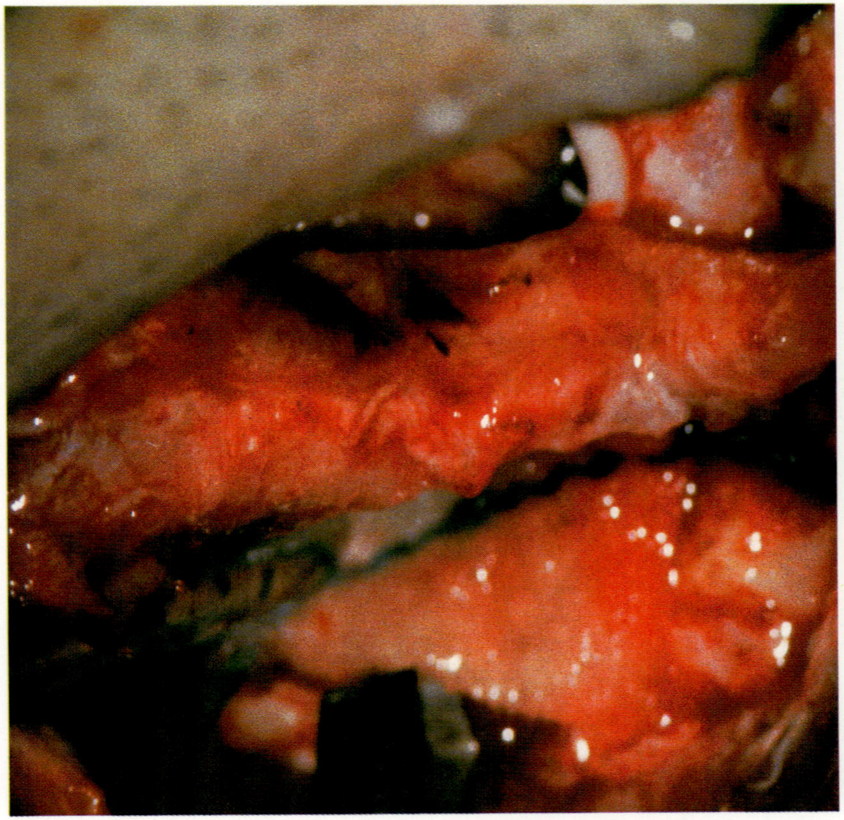

54

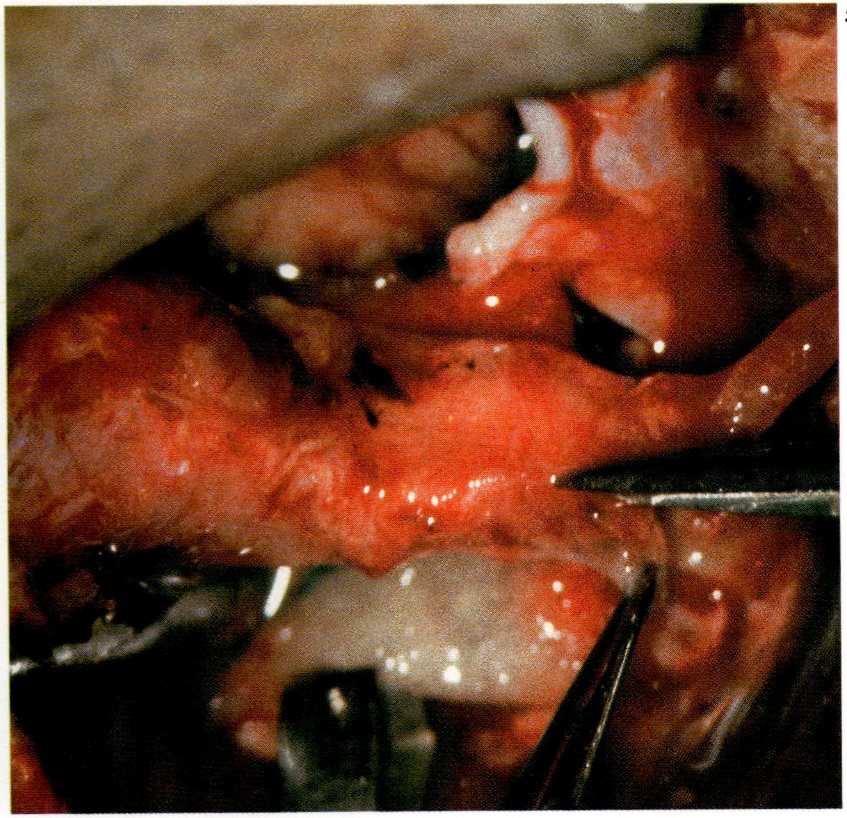

53 A pattie has been placed over the clamped cortical artery and the dural defect. The superficial temporal artery pedicle is brought across the centre of the field.

54 The superficial temporal artery is further mobilised under the microscope. The extra magnification allows specific identification and coagulation of small branches. Close dissection to the artery is possible without damaging its wall.

55

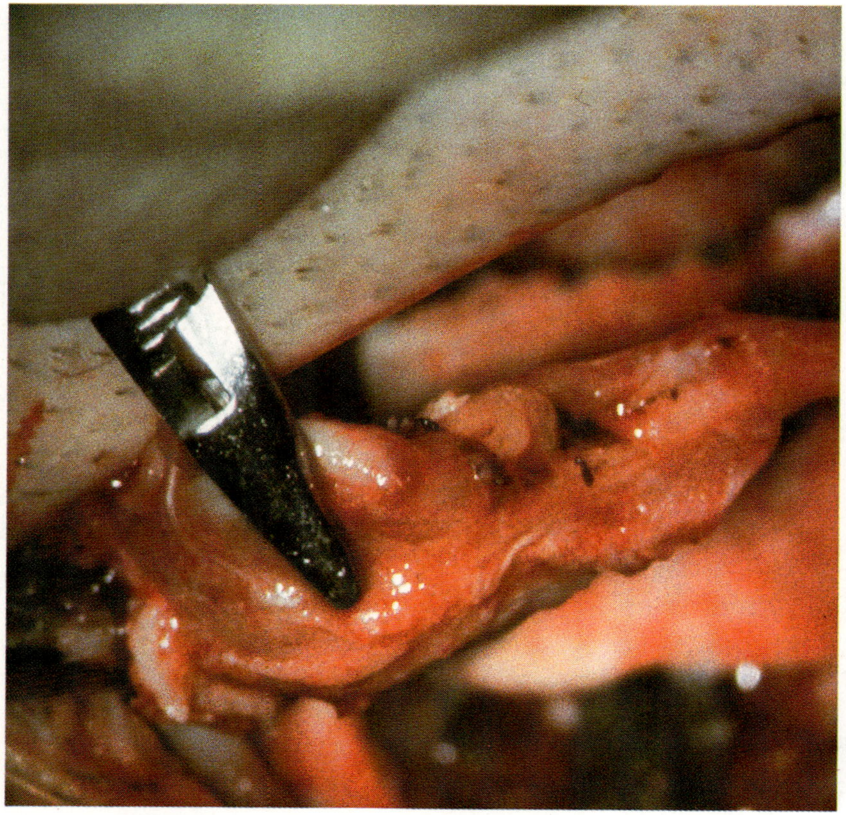

55 A section of superficial temporal artery at the proximal end of the wound has been isolated and a ¾″ bulldog clamp is being placed across its proximal end. The bulldog is chosen to have just enough pressure to occlude the artery without damaging its wall.

56

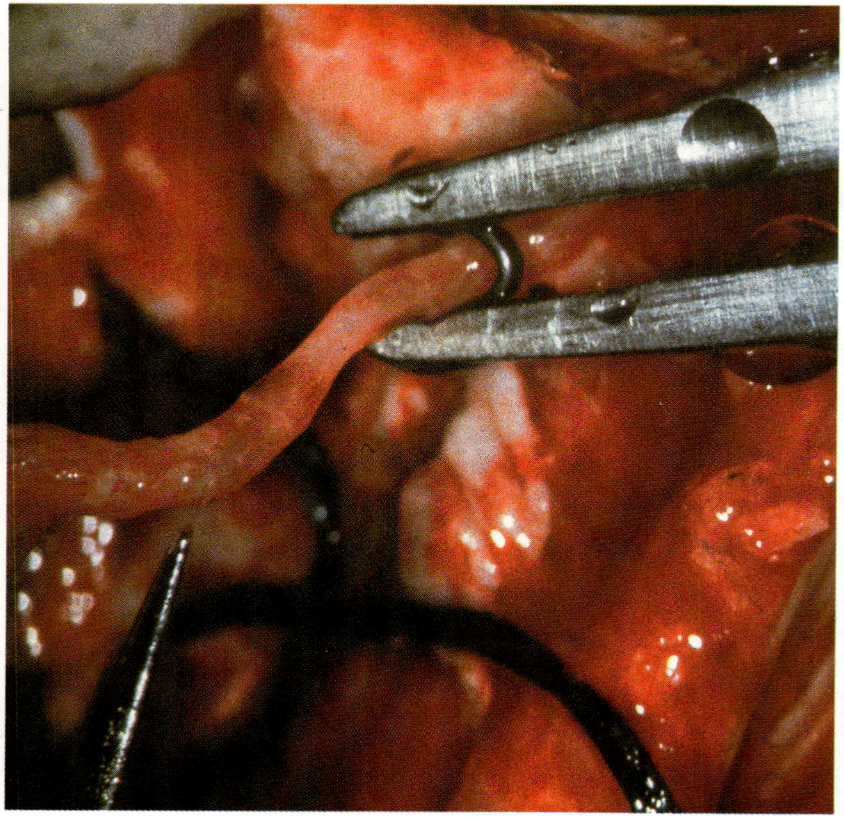

56 A silver clip is applied to the distal end of the vessel.

57

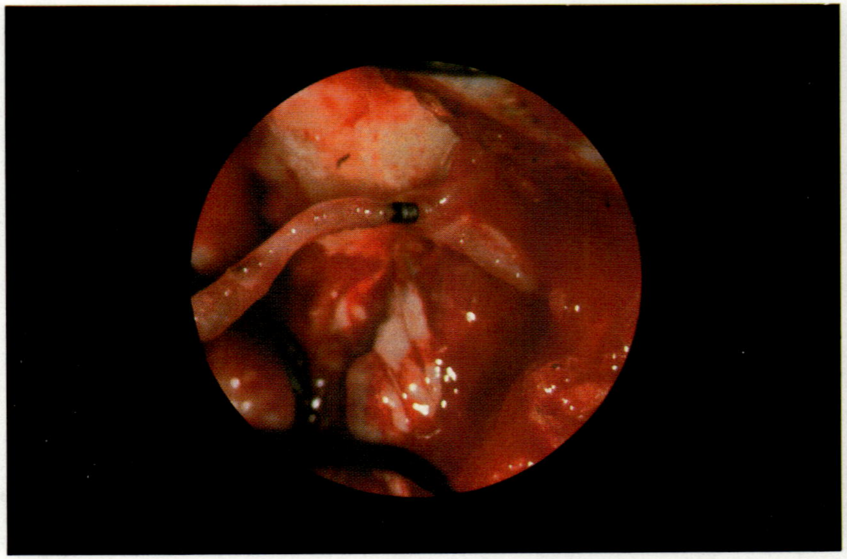

58

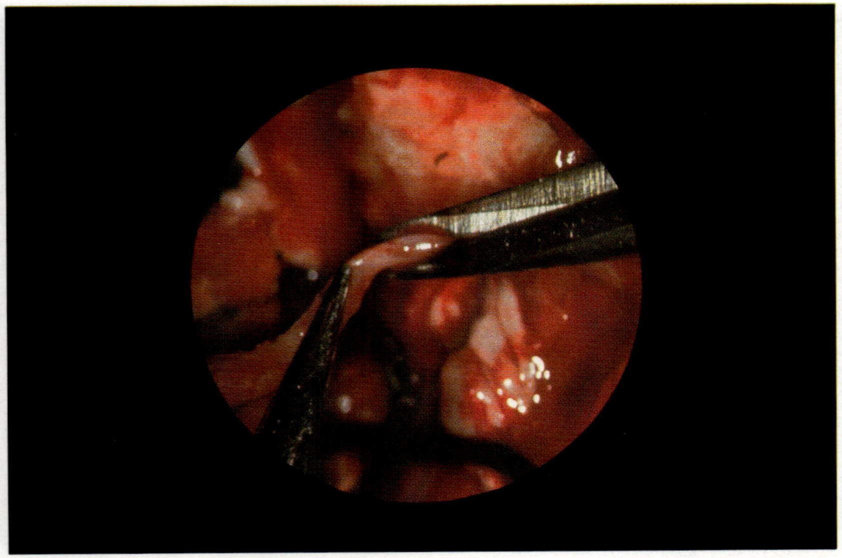

57 The clip is closed and the vessel is ready for division.

58 The vessel is divided obliquely to approximately match the elliptical incision in the cortical vessel.

59 Completion of the division.

59

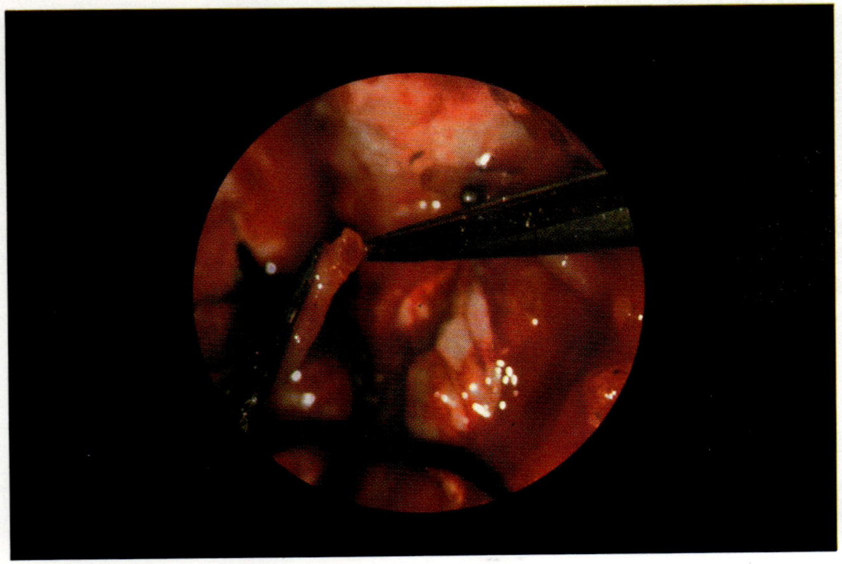

The anastomosis

60

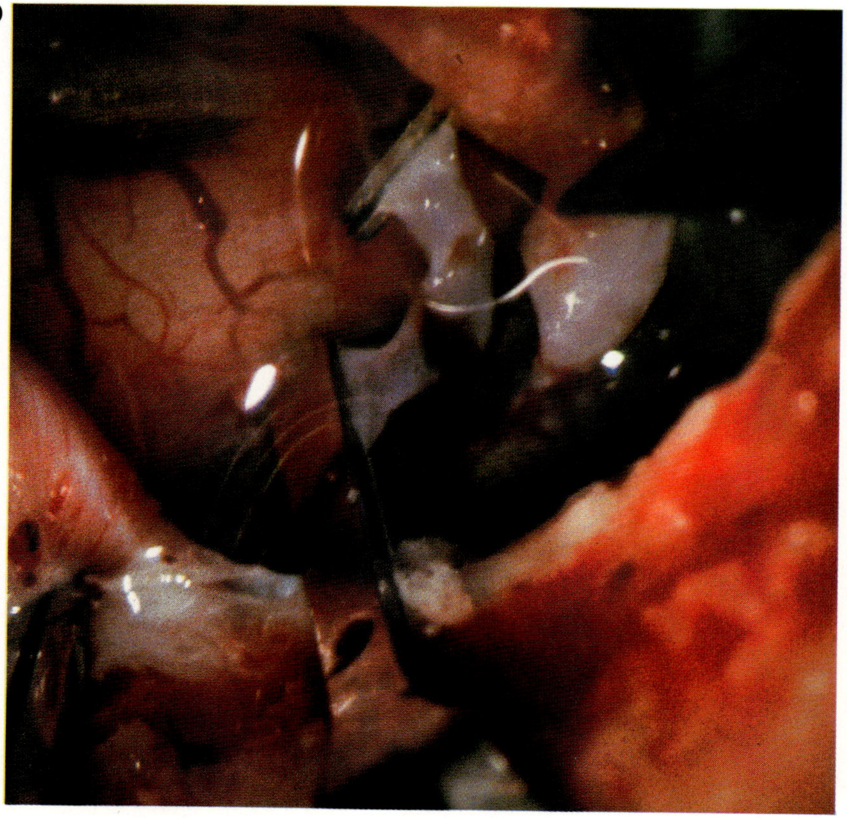

61

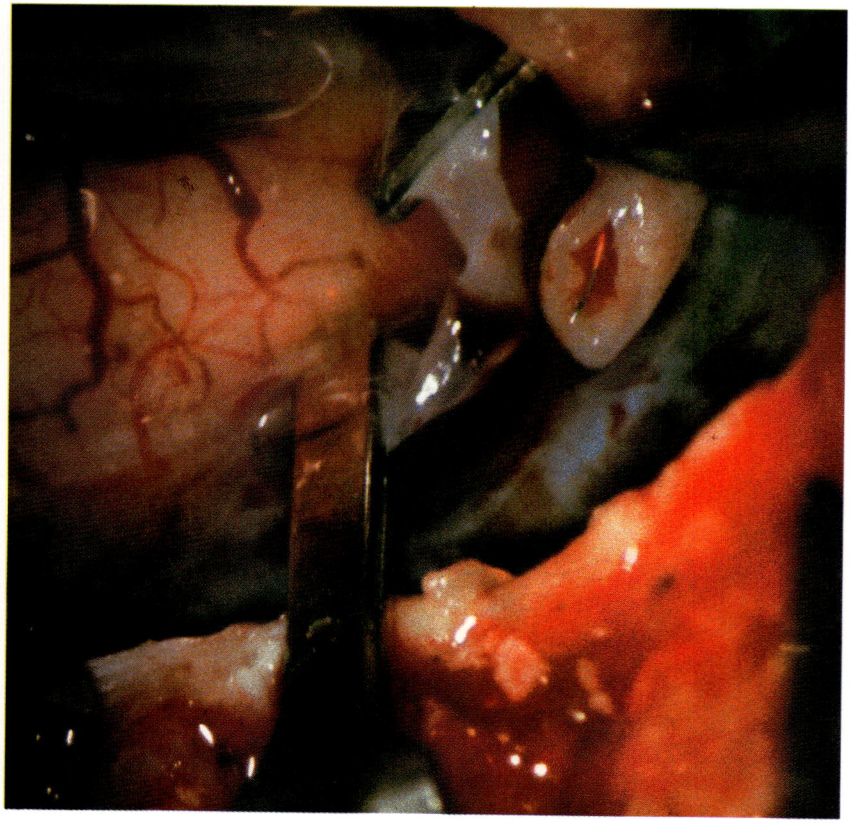

60 The microscope is re-focused on the cortical vessel and the divided superficial temporal artery is brought down alongside it. At this stage the superficial temporal artery orifice may need to be lengthened or redivided to match the cortical vessel. Additional strands of adventitia over the distal 5 mm or 6 mm are trimmed away. The pedicle is placed so that the artery is not under tension during suture and there is no twist along its axis. The size of the anastomosis is in the region of 3 mm. The end-to-side union allows blood from the scalp artery to pass both proximally and distally in the middle cerebral branch.

61 The first of the interrupted sutures is being placed, starting in the scalp artery. The first stitch is usually placed on the side away from the surgeon, subsequent sutures being placed on either side of it, progressing around to the front. With a freely mobile pedicle, this order is not necessarily followed, because the anastomosis can be easily turned from side to side allowing access to stitches in the far corner, even at a later stage.

62

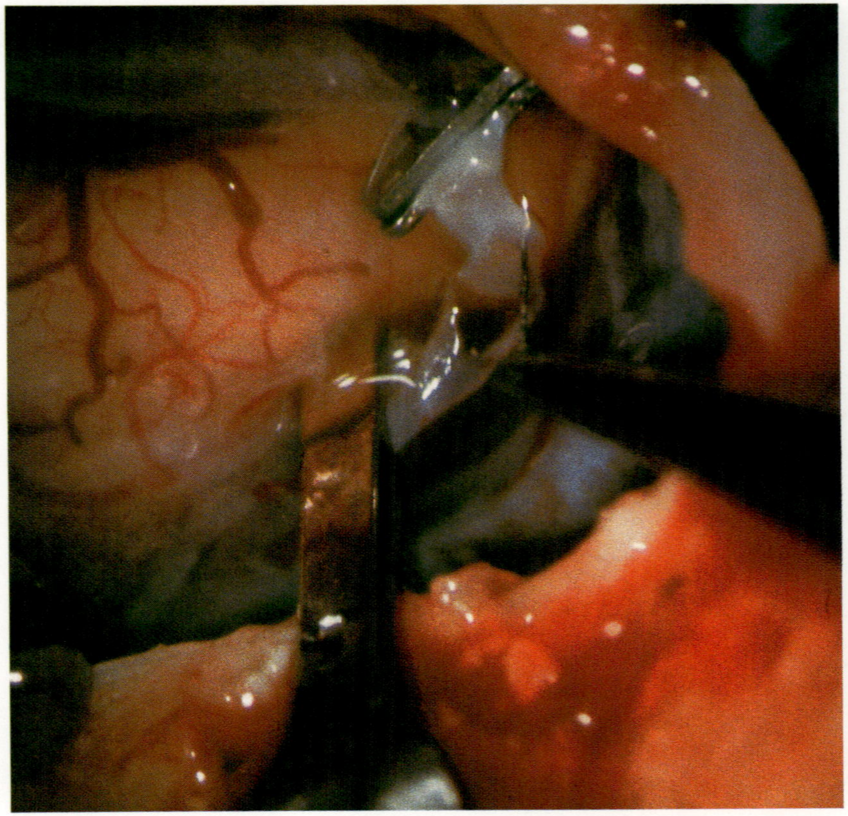

62 The needle has been drawn through the scalp artery and reversed. It is inserted into the appropriate site in the cortical vessel.

63

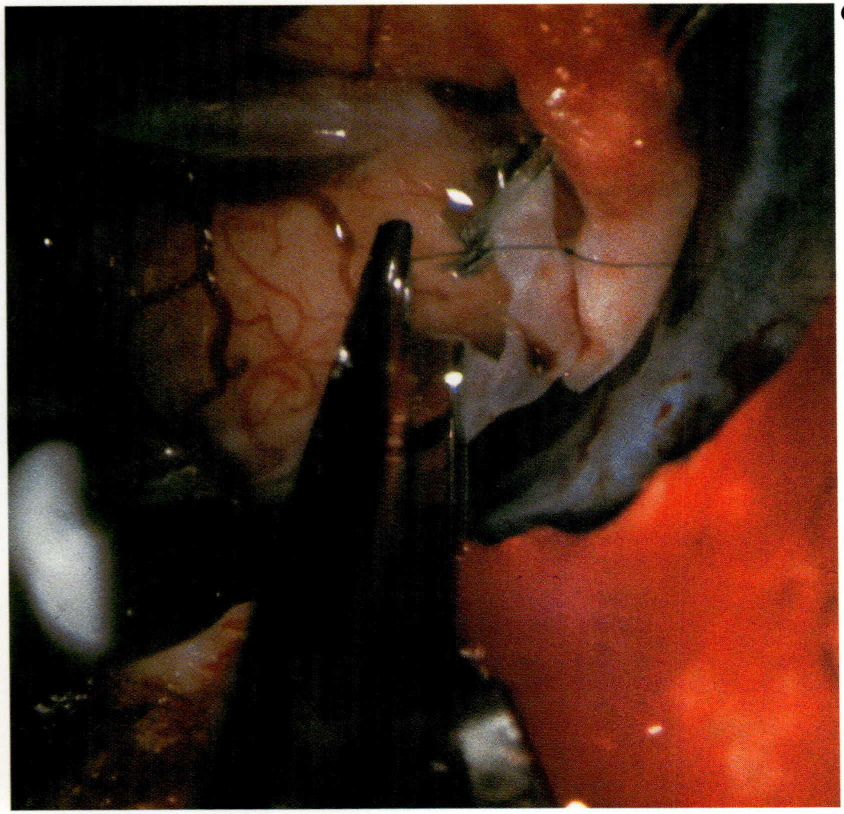

63 The first suture is tied and serves to approximate the two arteries.

64

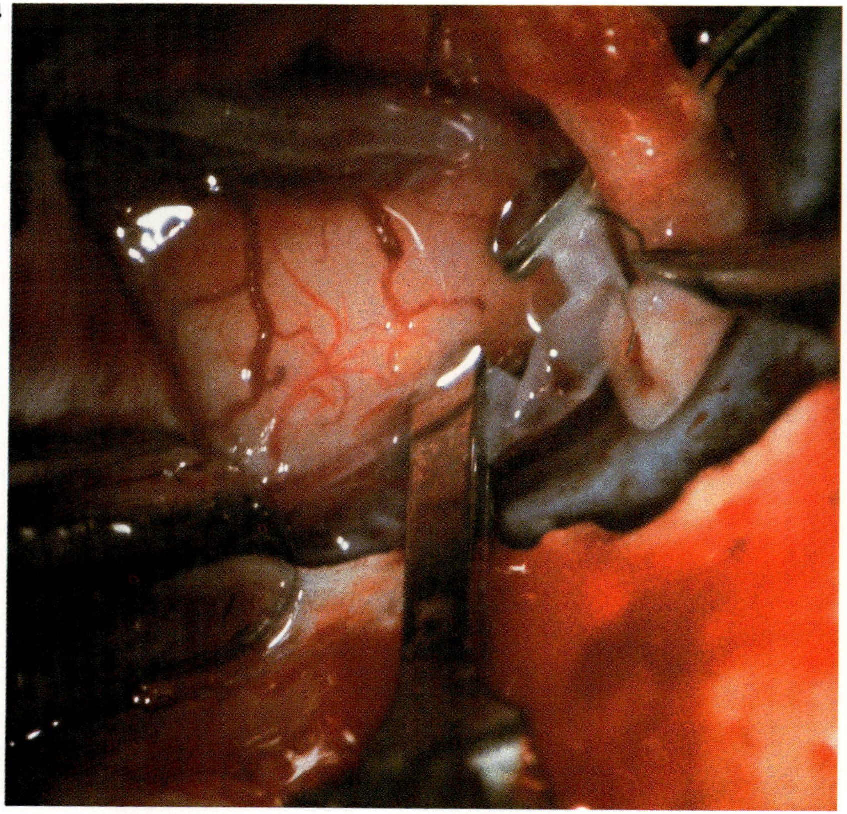

65

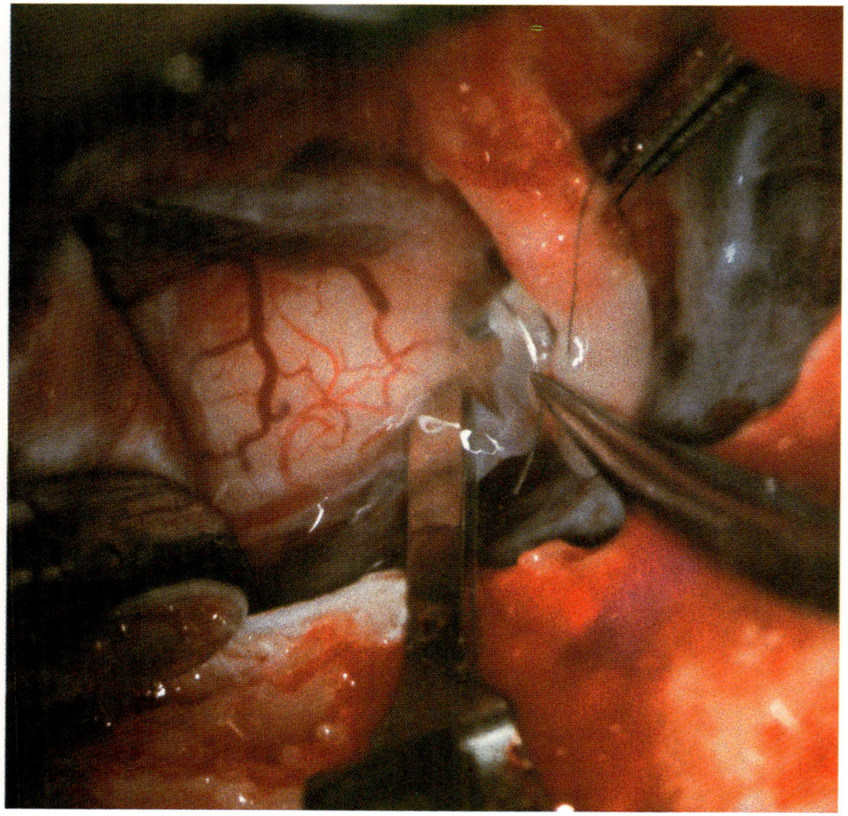

64 The second suture on this occasion is in the angle of each arteriotomy.

65 The needle is reversed and is passed through the angle of the cortical vessel. Under this magnification a fine 10/0 monofilament nylon is not easily seen when it is out of focus: the portion entering the scalp artery can be identified.

66

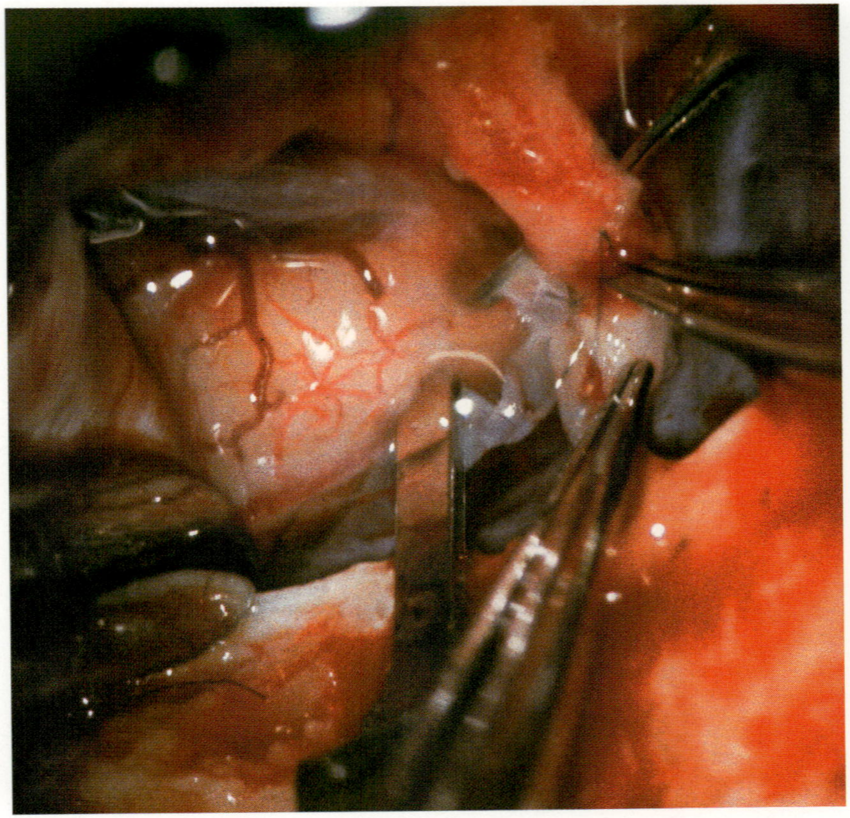

66 The commencement of the third stitch. The knot of the second is visible in the angle between the vessels.

67

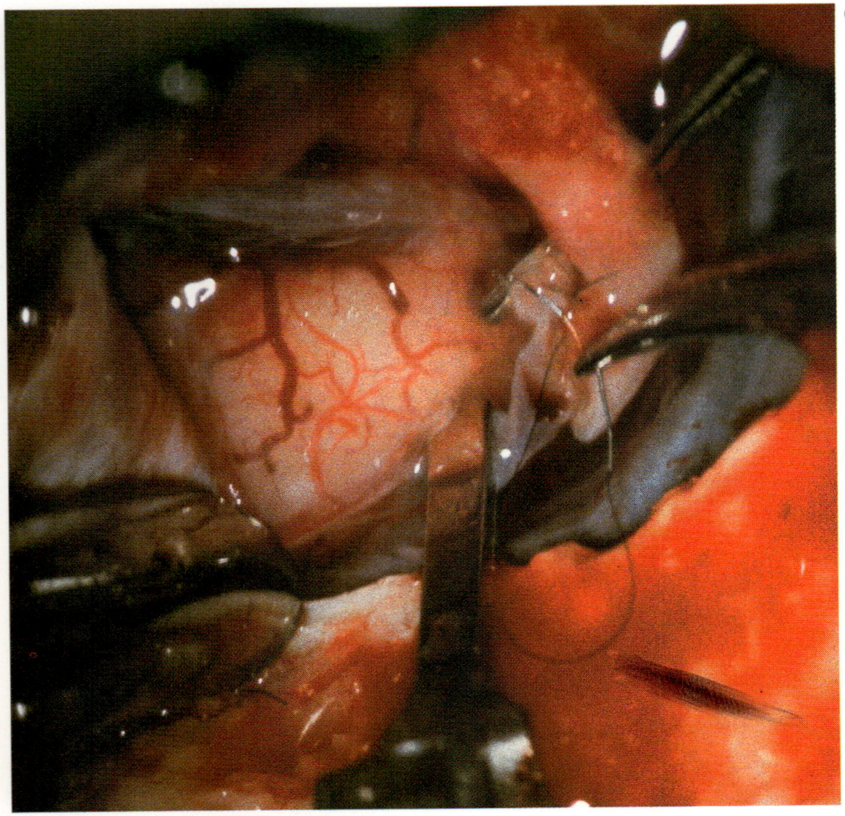

67 Needle reversed and placed in the cortical vessel for third stitch of anastomosis.

68

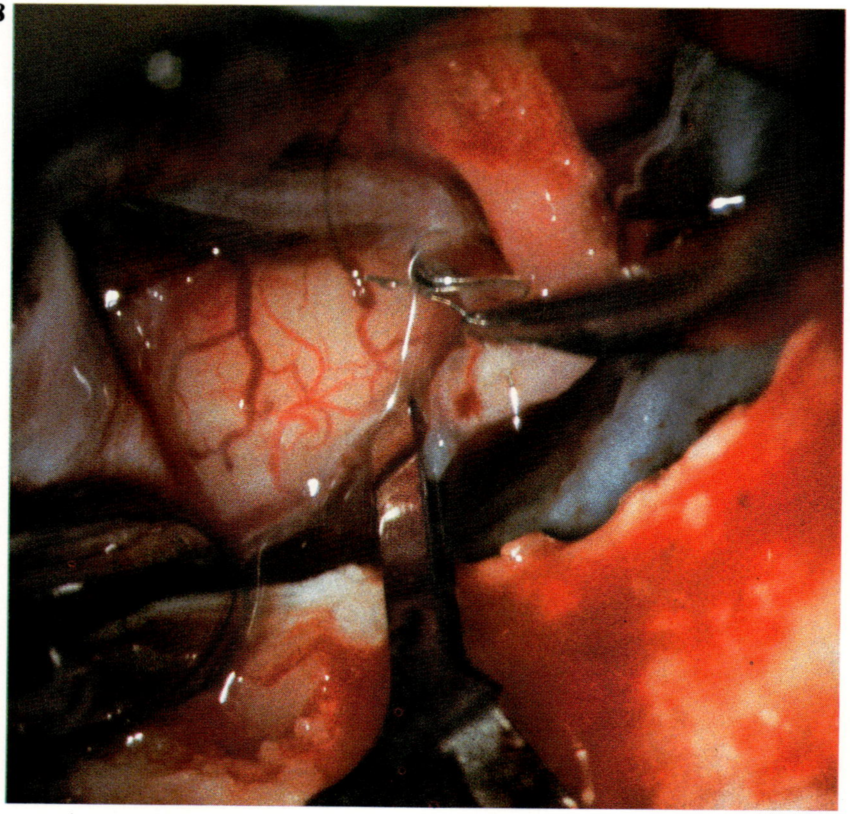

68 The two vessels are closely and accurately applied and at this stage the direction of suture and the order is based on ease of application. In this photograph a stitch is being inserted through both vessels at the same time, the needle passing first through the cortical vessel.

69

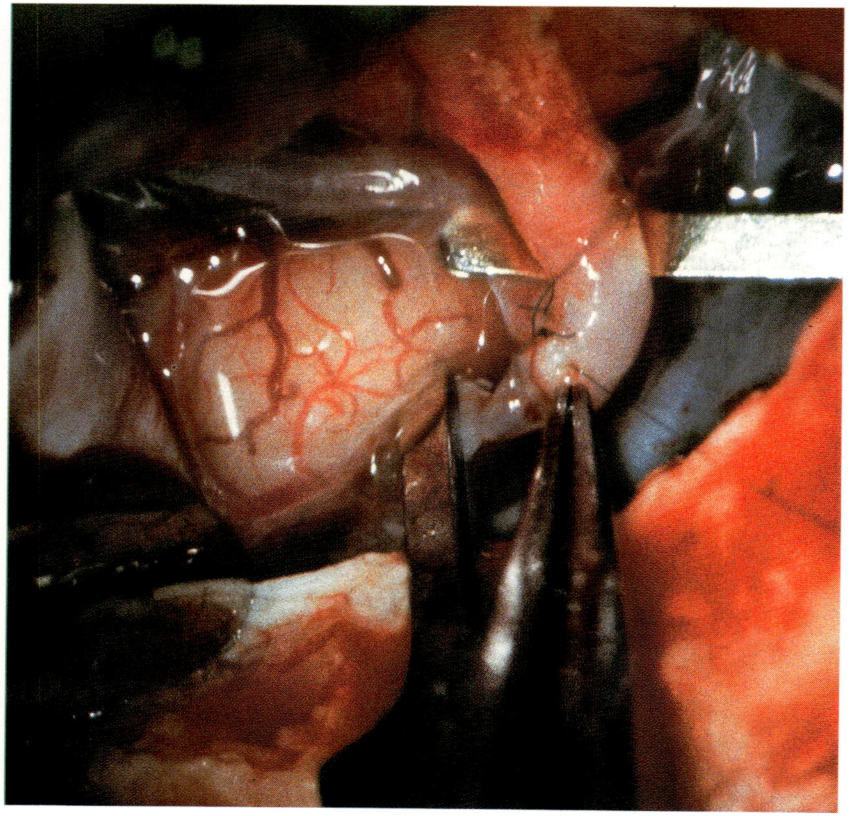

69 The suture is drawn through the two vessel walls – following removal of the needle in the previous photograph.

70

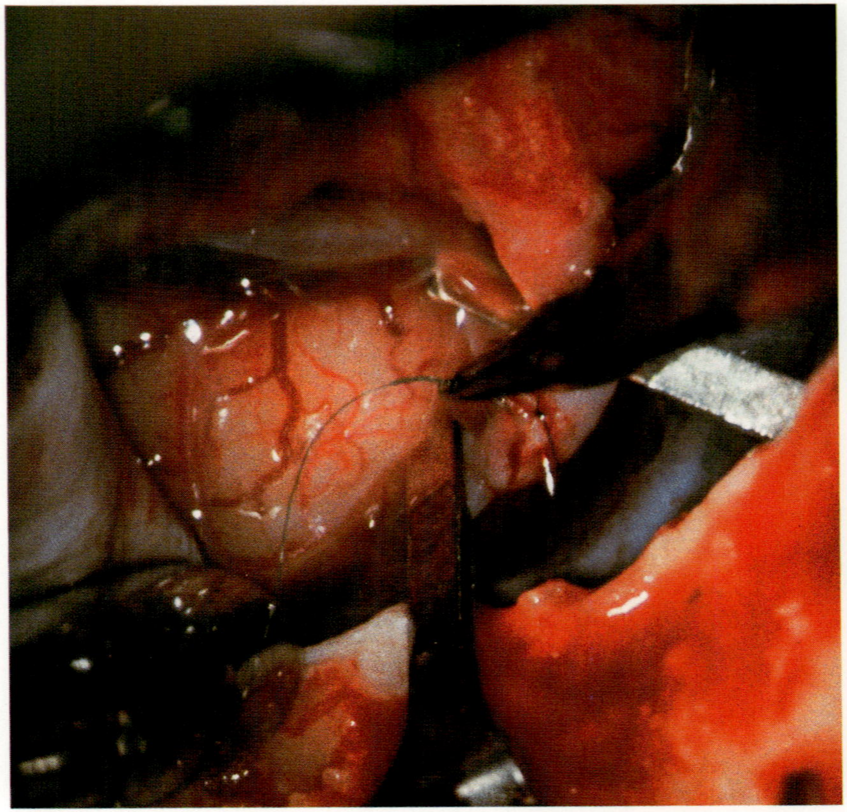

71

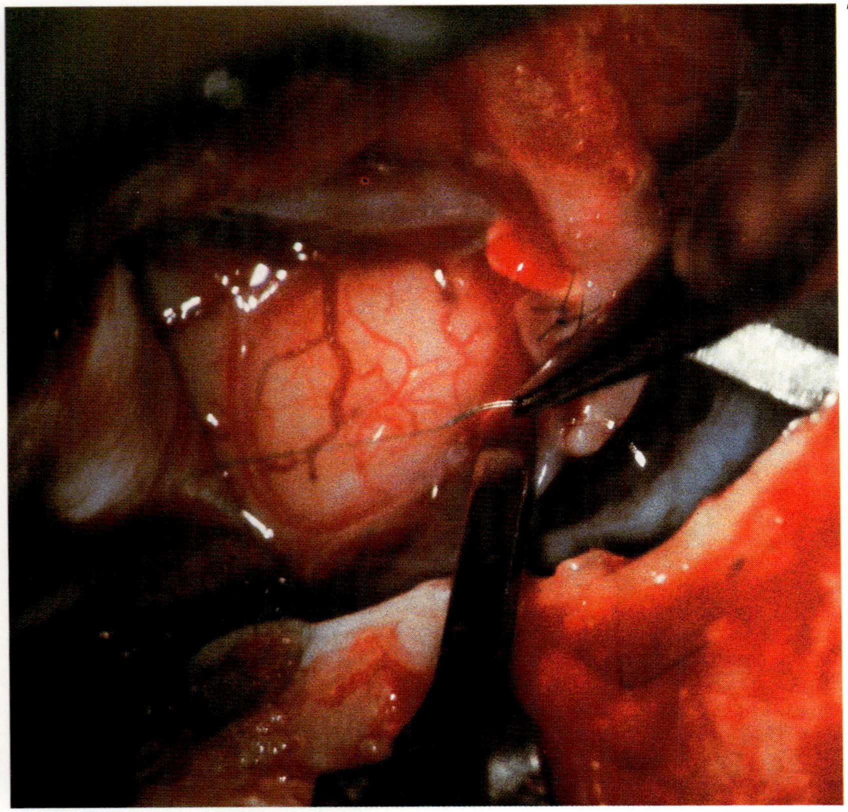

70 **The anastomosis in nearing the second corner and, in this case, the direction and placement of the needle is again from the cortical to the scalp vessel.**

71 **Another suture placed close to the second corner.**

72

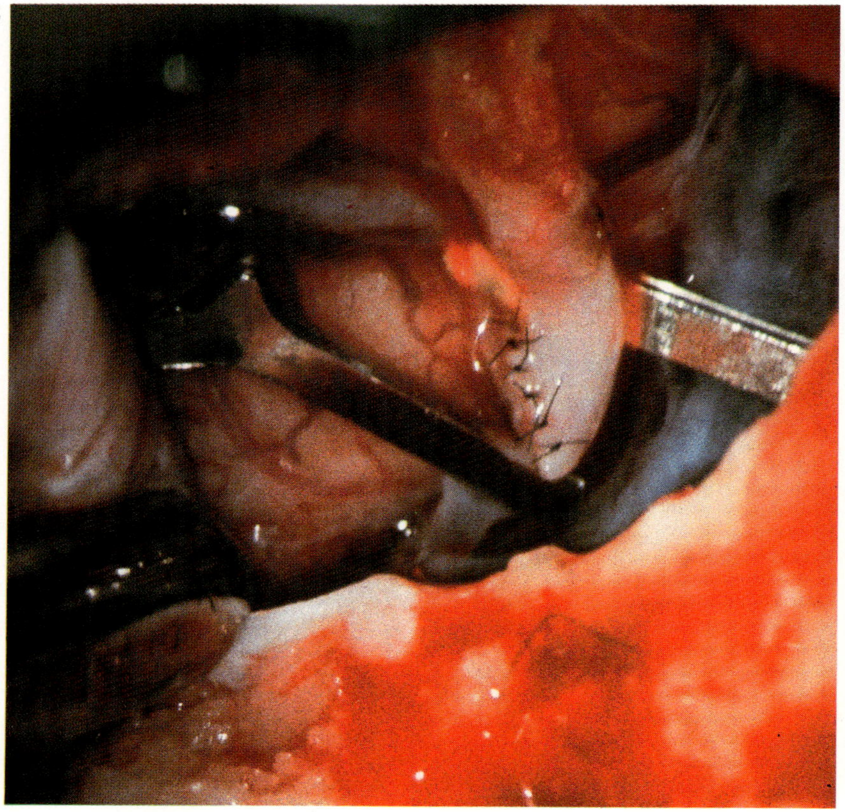

72 **The first side of the anastomosis is near completion.**

73

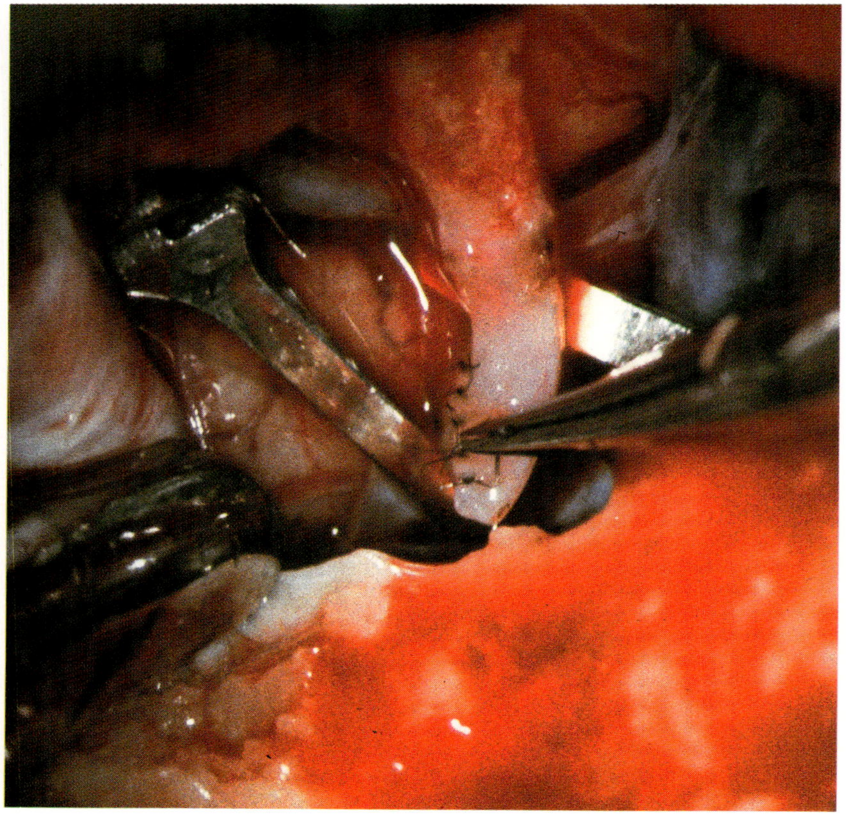

73 **A corner suture, placed first in the scalp vessel.**

74

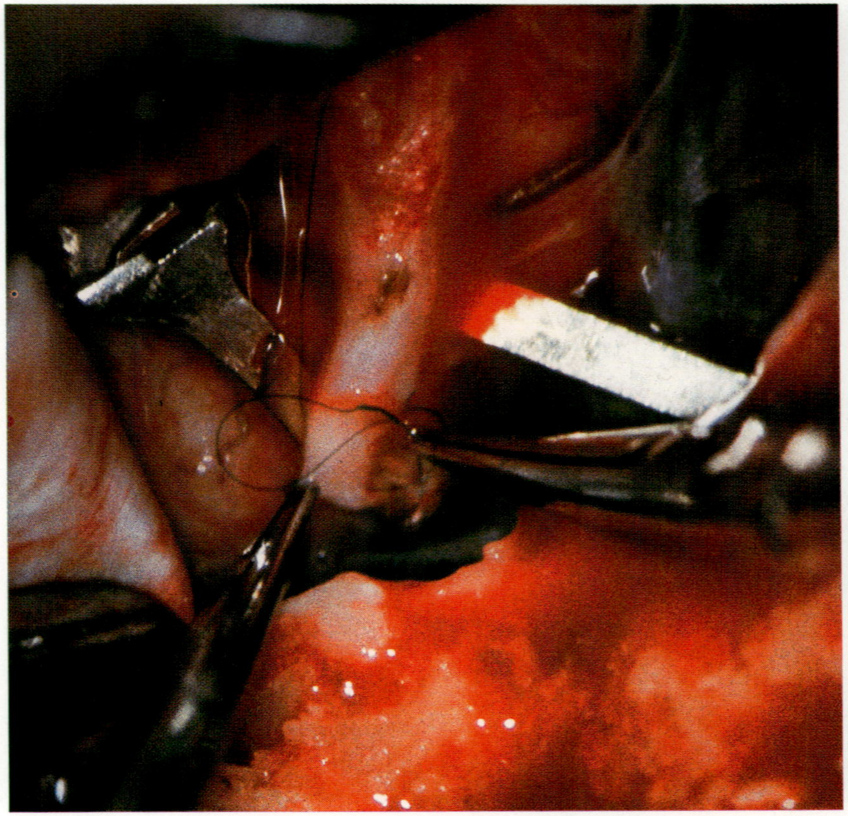

74 The corner suture placed in the cortical vessel. As with the early sutures the two manoeuvres shown in this and the previous photograph are undertaken as separate stages, to ensure accurate picking up of the two vessel walls without adventitial inclusion in the suture line.

75

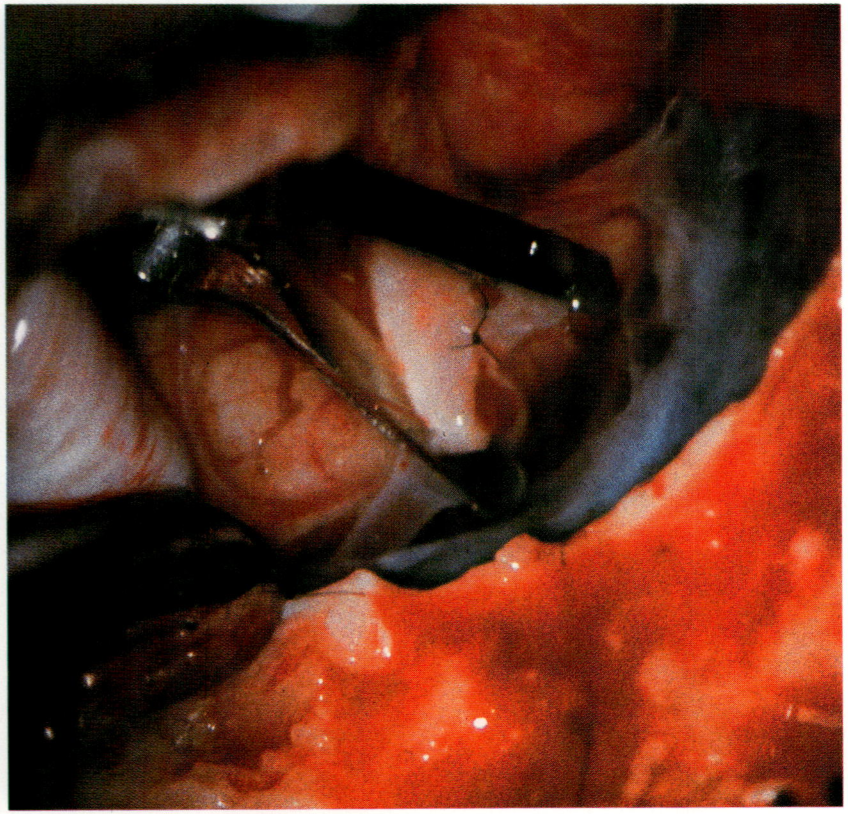

75 The second corner suture. It was decided at an early stage that it would be convenient to turn the anastomosis over to allow access to the second side. The upper clip on the cortical vessel has been rotated to bring into view the second half of the anastomosis. The first stitch of the anastomosis is seen from a different direction.

76

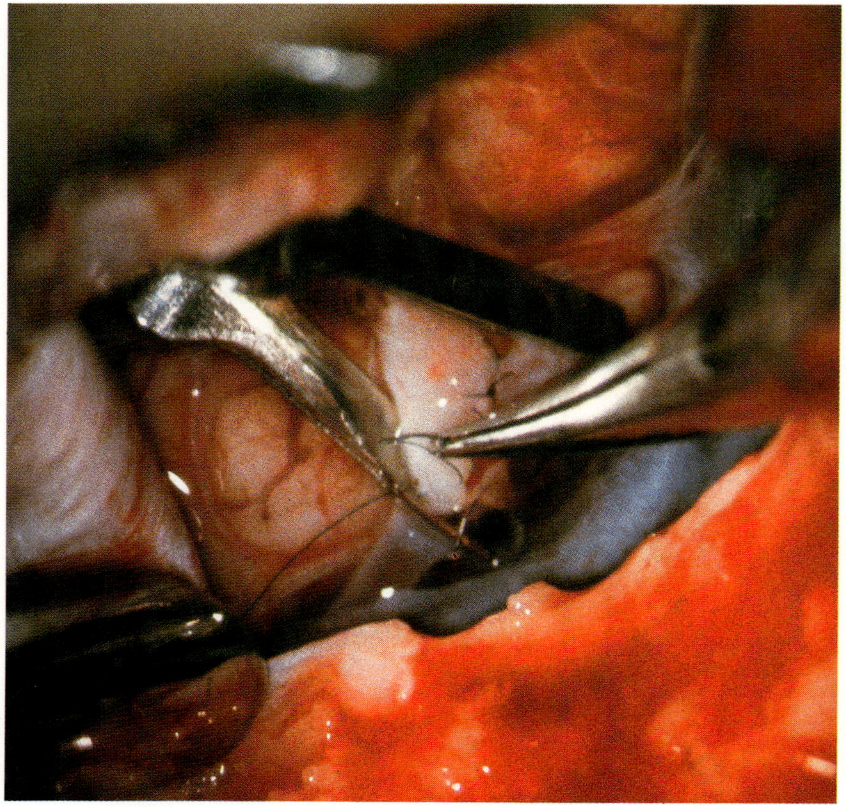

77

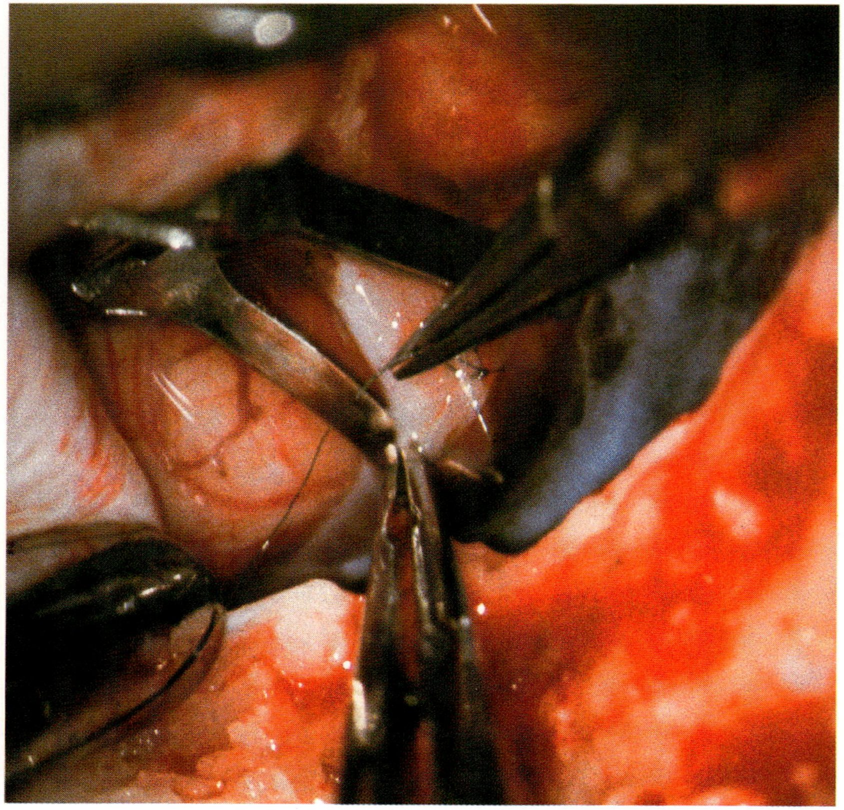

76 The placement of another corner stitch. It is again being undertaken in two stages, the first having been completed and the needle is being inserted into the cortical vessel. The suture is seen passing from the deep surface of the scalp vessel to the needle.

77 Further stitches have been applied to the second side of the anastomosis and another three stitches are required. With the close apposition of the two vessels, it is possible to accurately pass the needle through both vessels at once without fear of misplacement.

78

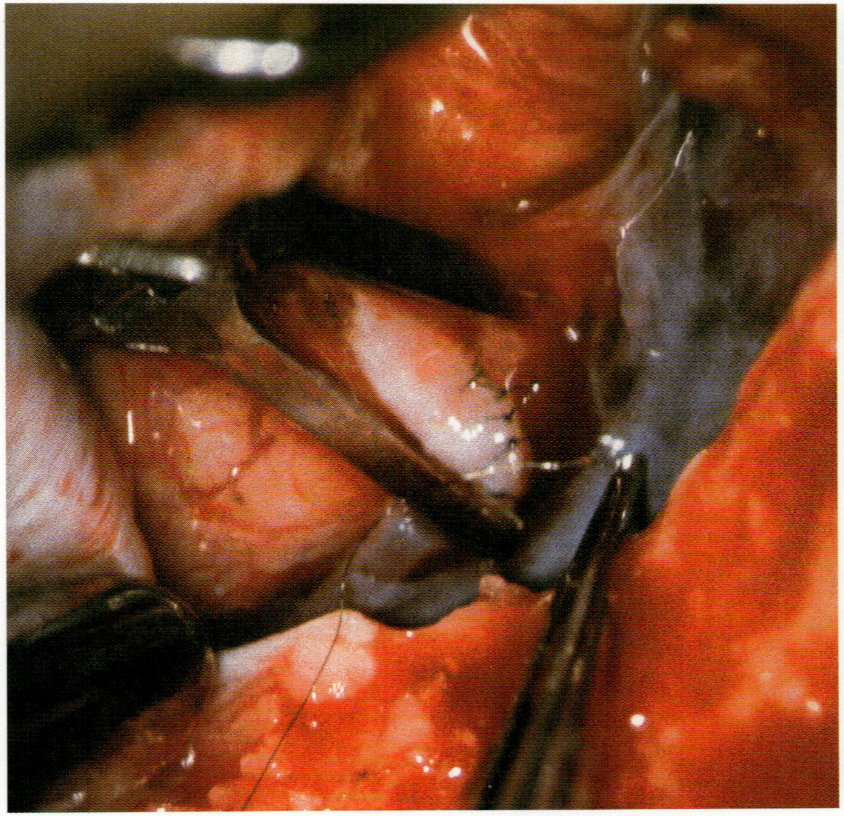

79

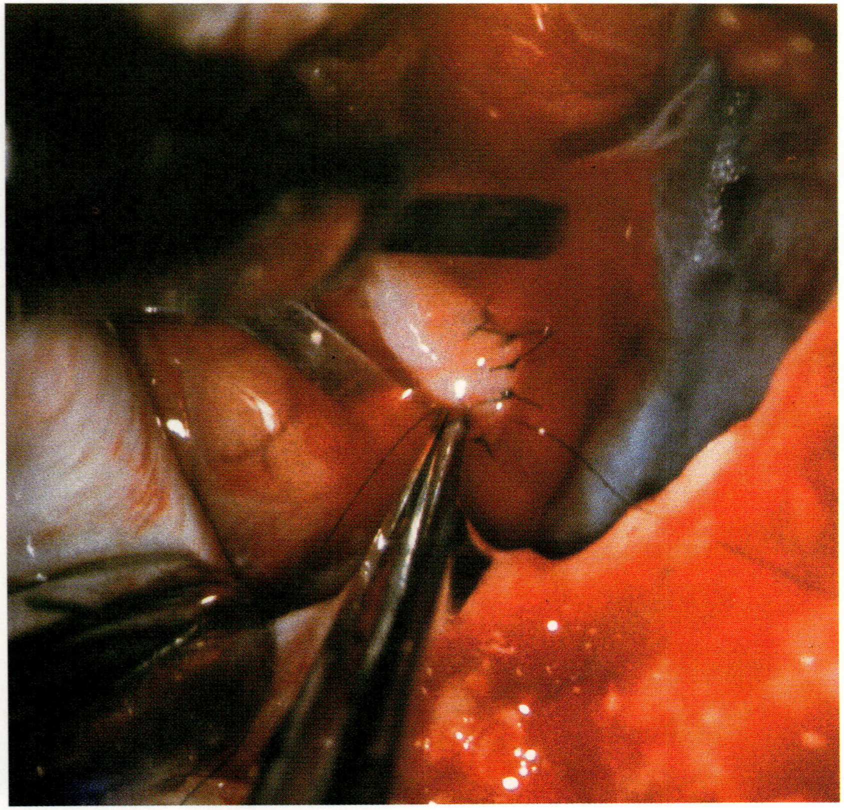

78 Placement of the final suture from the cortical to the scalp vessel. The suture is left in place but not tied at this stage.

79 The clip on the cortical vessel at the upper end of the photograph is being temporarily released and blood is seen leaking from the last unsutured portion of the anastomosis, confirming free-flow from this end of the cortical vessel.

80

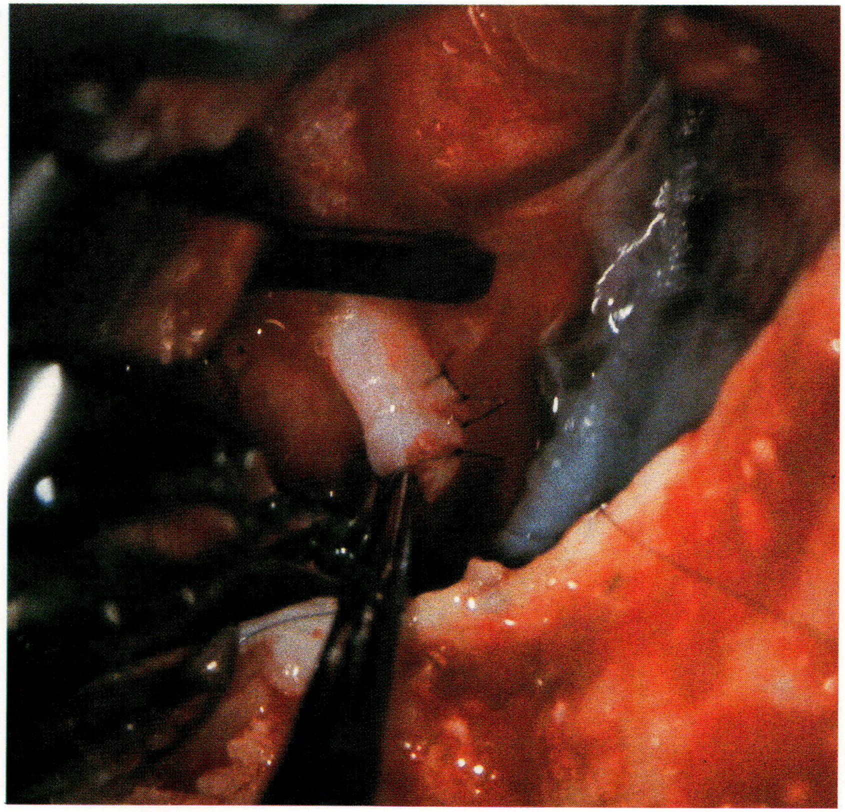

81

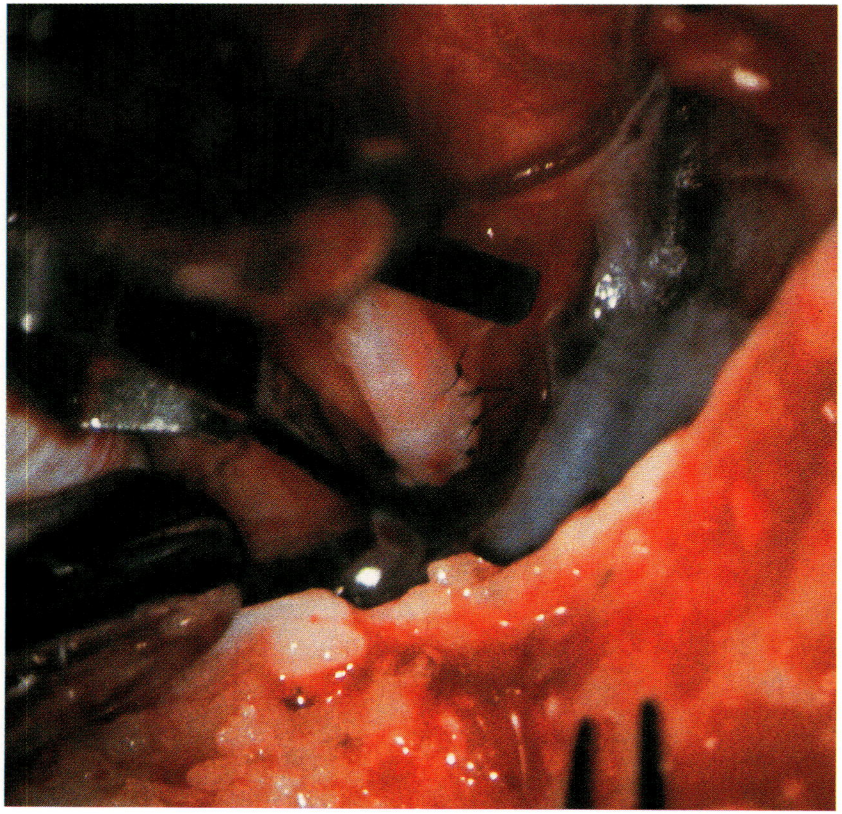

80 The clip applicator applied to the lower clip. The scalp artery is being steadied by a watchmaker forceps applied to its adventitia. Free-flow was obtained from this end of the anastomosis, together with pulsatile flow when temporarily releasing the bulldog clip on the scalp artery.

81 The final stitch has been tied and the applicator reapplied to release the upper cortical clip.

82

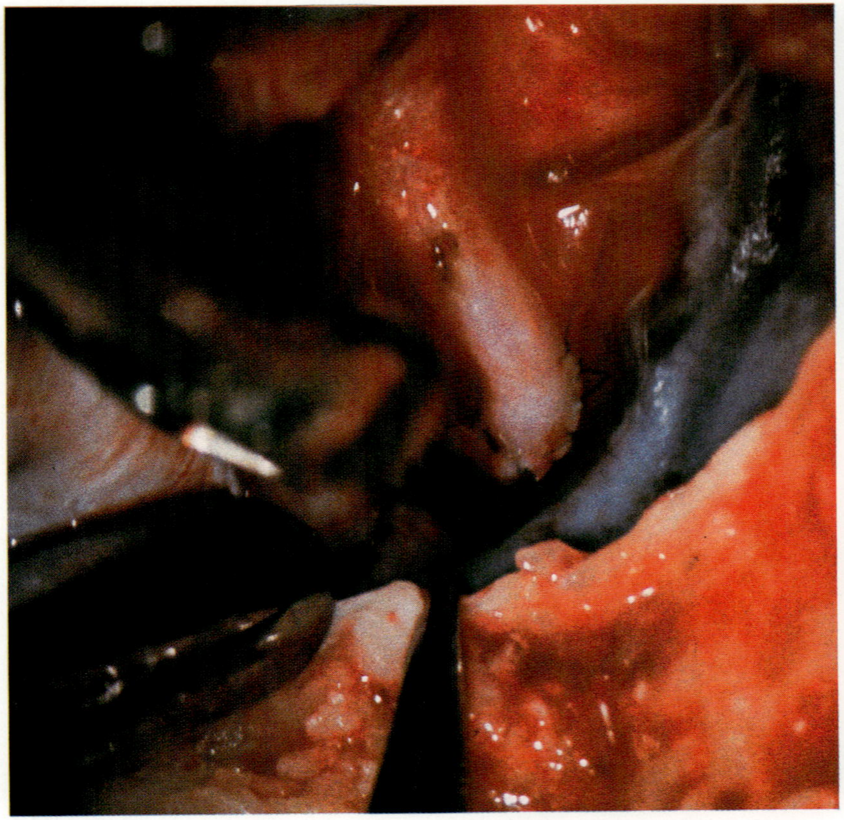

82 The upper clip has been removed and there is no leakage from the anastomosis. The lower clip is being removed.

83

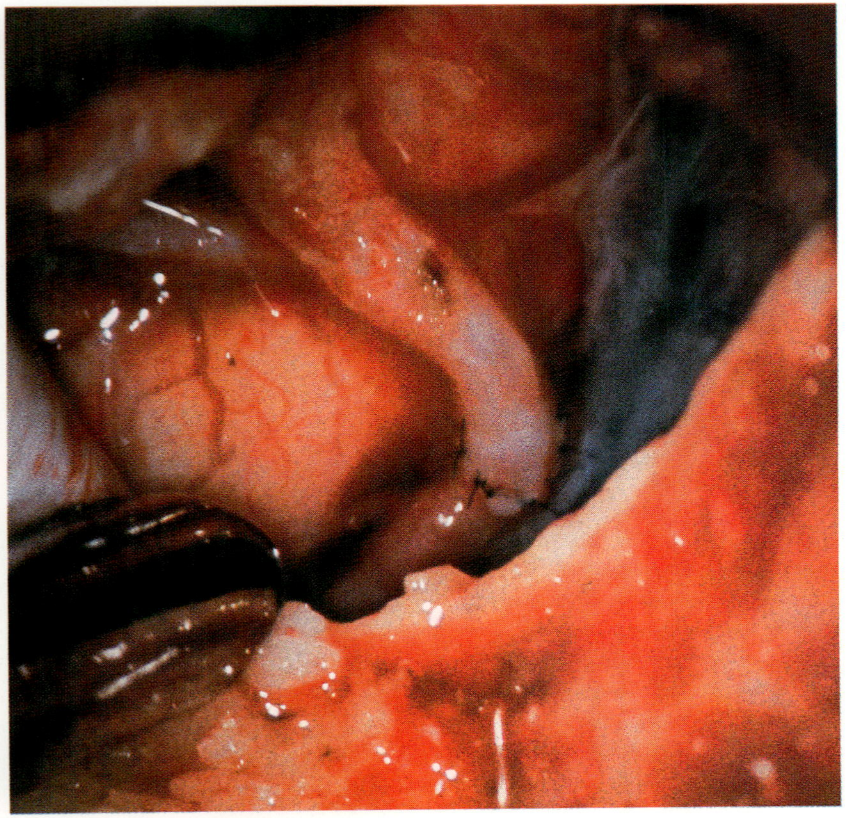

83 Both clips removed from the cortical artery. Some bleeding from the pedicle is present, the cortical arteries are adequately filled. At this stage it is important to confirm patency by gently lifting the scalp vessel over a watchmaker forceps, pulsation being seen in the partly occluded segment. Alternately, gently empty the blood from 6 mm or 7 mm of the scalp artery by using two watchmaker forceps. The first is gently closed and the second is used to squeeze the blood out of the segment: refilling on release of the forceps confirms flow. *This procedure must be carried out with great care to avoid damage to the intima.*

84

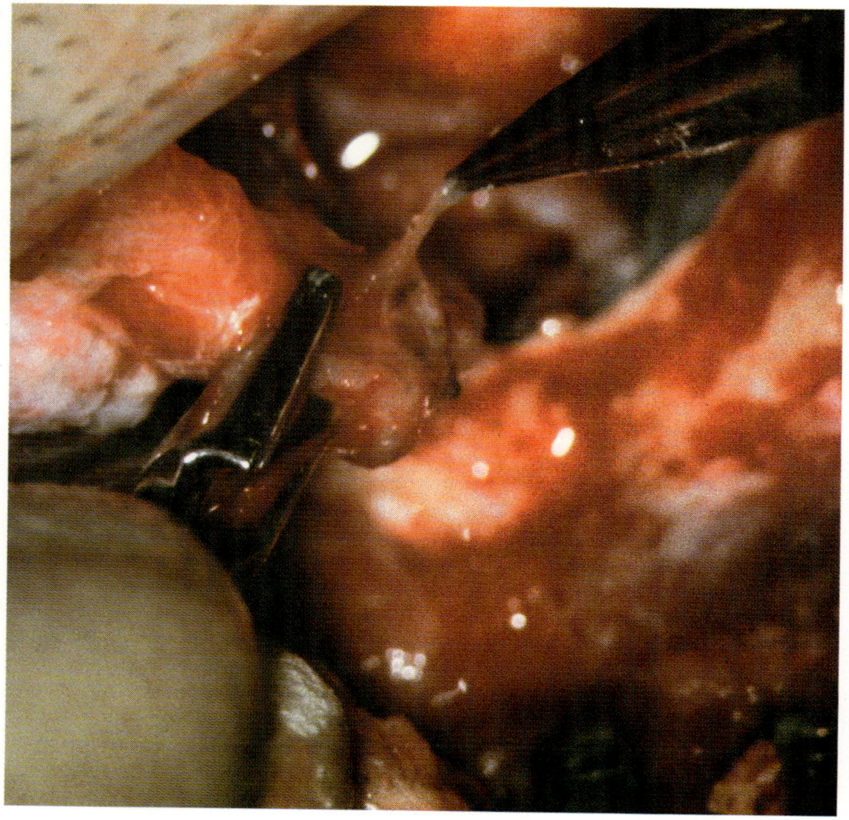

84 Bulldog clips being removed from the scalp pedicle.

85

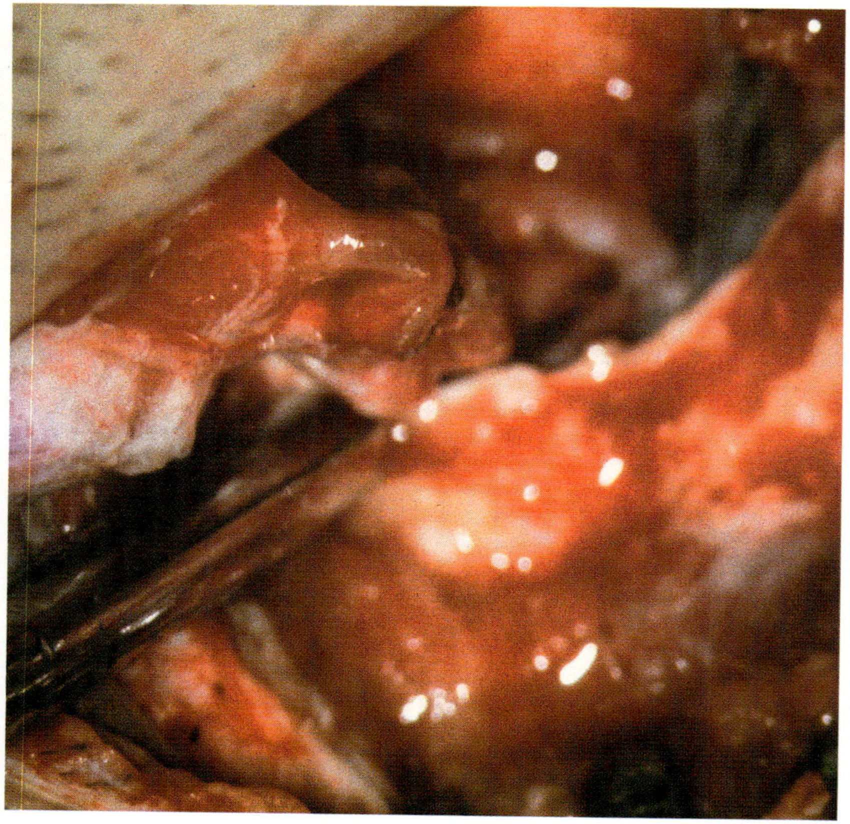

85 After bulldog clip removal the clamped length of scalp vessel is seen to be fully dilated.

86

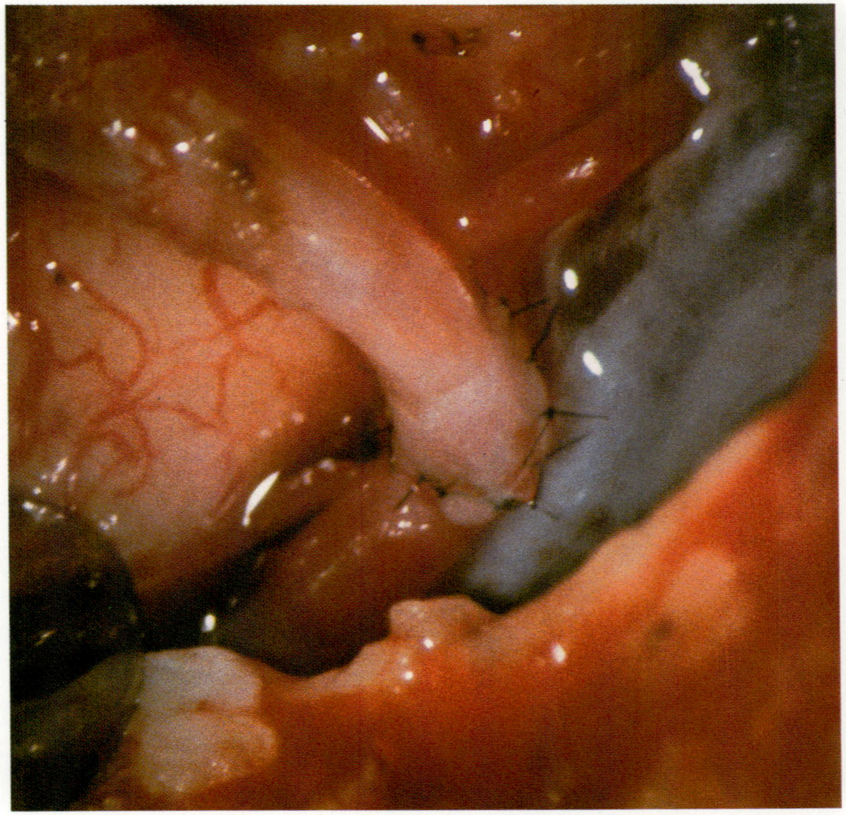

87

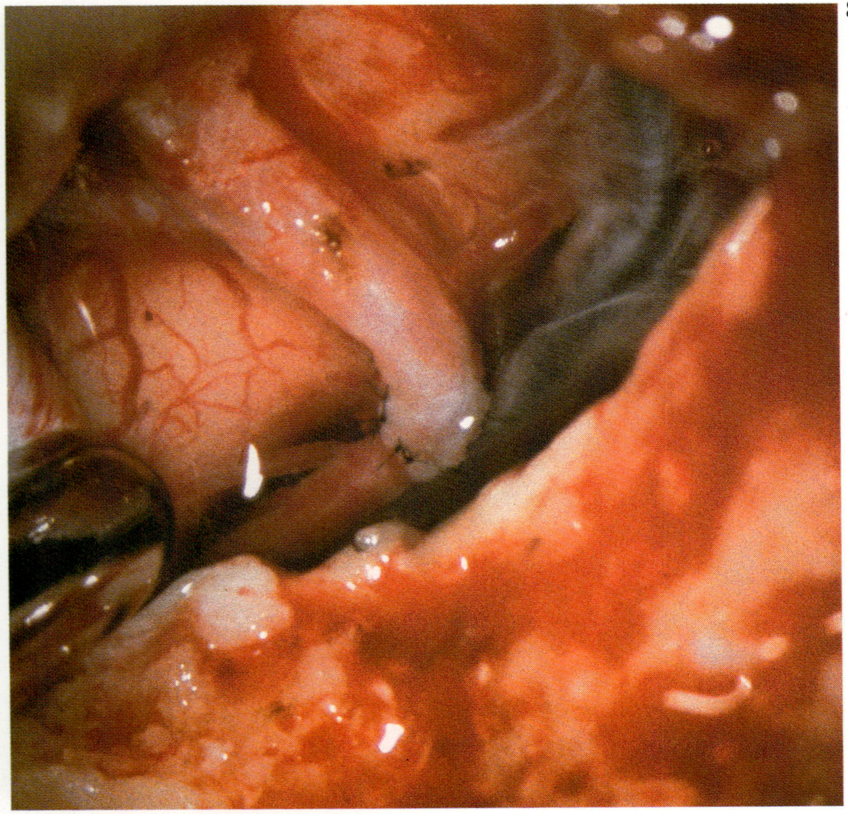

86 Haemostasis is established and the cortical vessel at each end of the anastomosis is fully expanded. Occasional areas of spasm at sites of clipping can be abolished by very gentle pressure across the cortical vessel with the tips of a watchmaker forceps.

87 Anastomosis at a lower magnification.

Dural closure

88

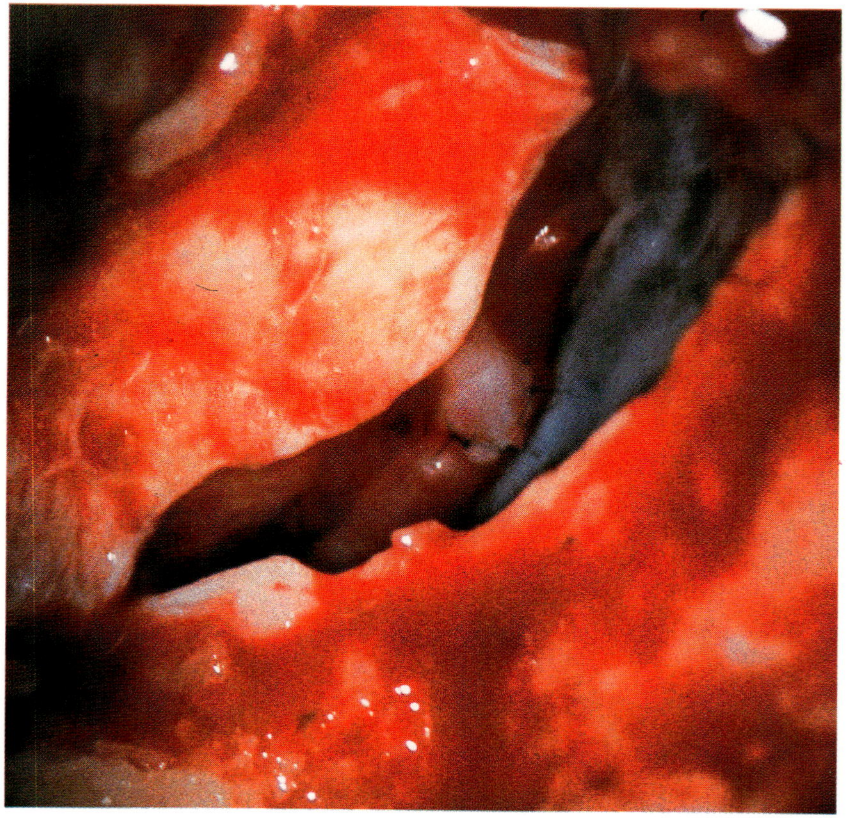

88 Dural flap being turned back.

89

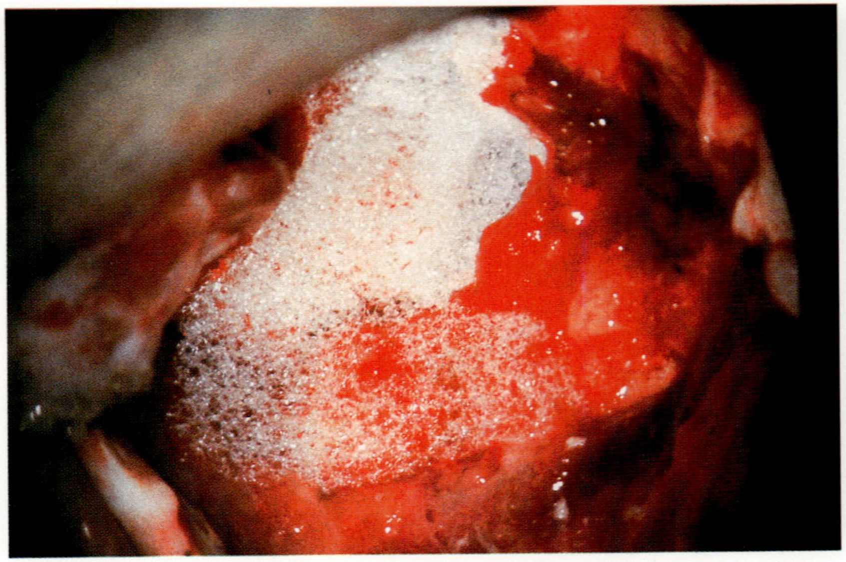

90

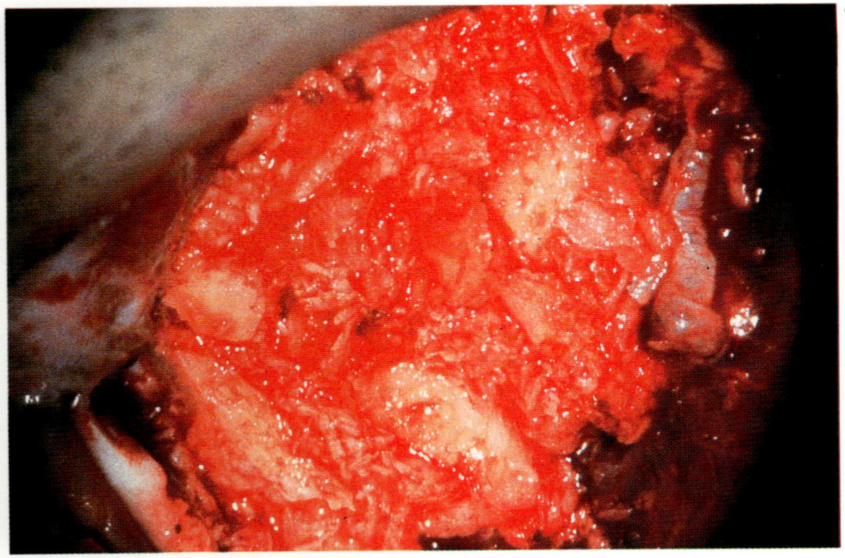

91

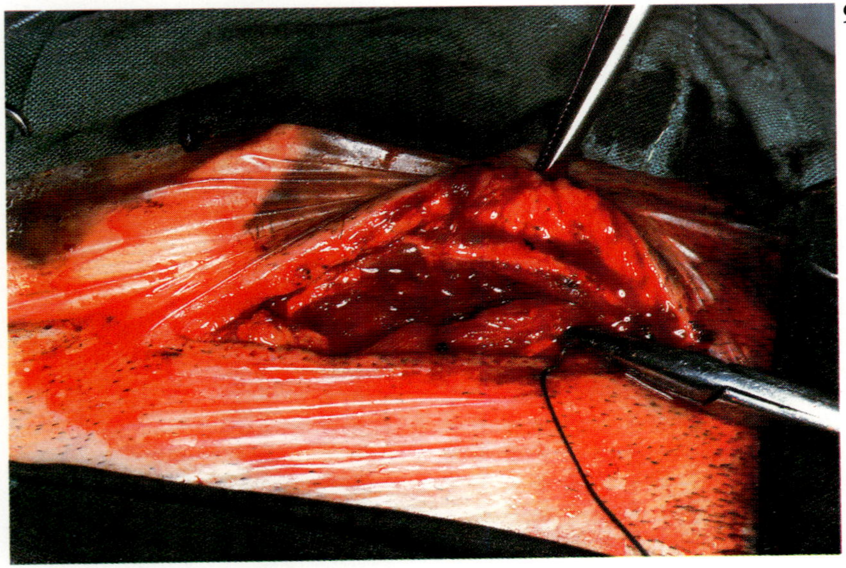

89 Single layer of gel foam placed over dural flap.

90 Bone filings replaced within bony defect.

91 Gentle approximation of temporalis muscle with a single stitch.

Skin closure and application of dressing

92
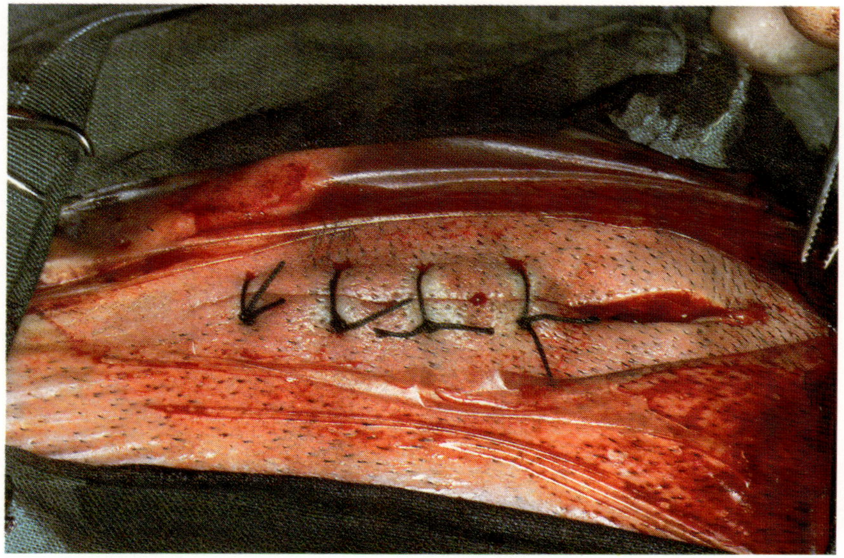

92 Skin closure without drainage.

93
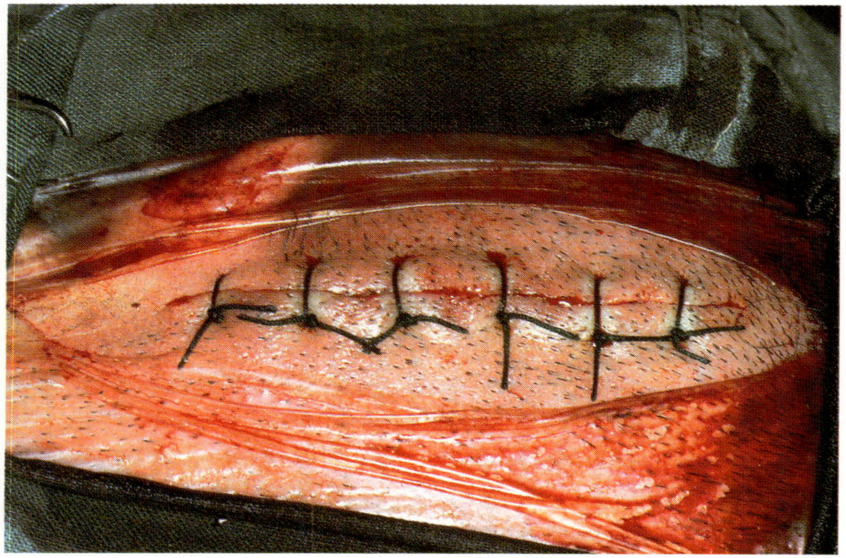

93 Skin closure completed.

94

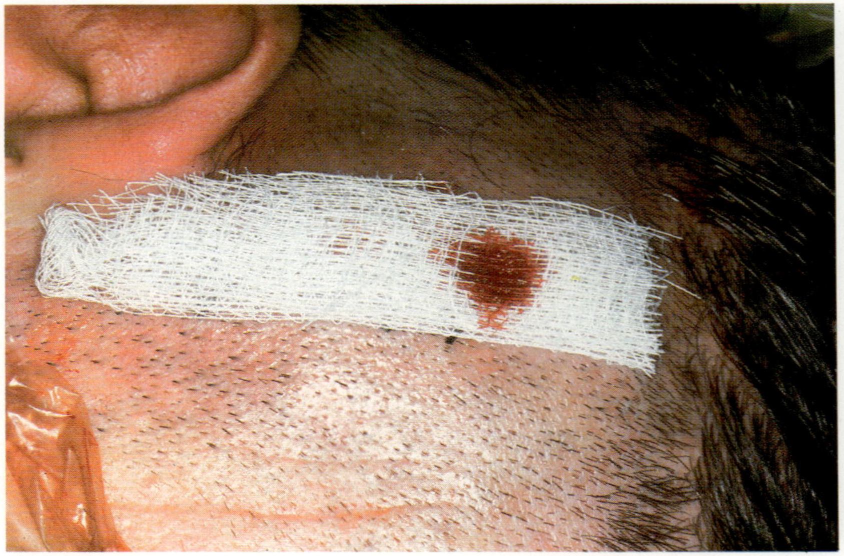

94 Light dressing applied.

95

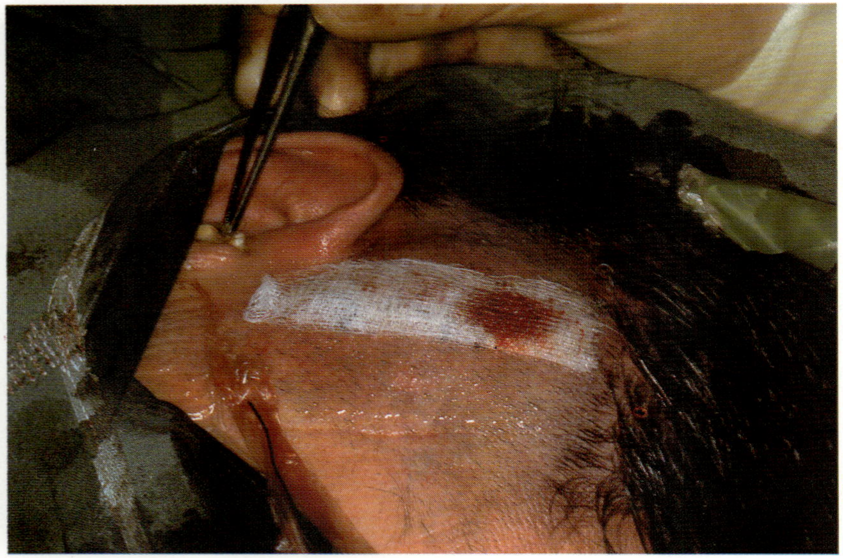

95 The dressing is stuck down with collodion, care being taken that the solution does not enter the patient's eye. The cotton wool ear-plug is removed. No head bandaging is required.

96

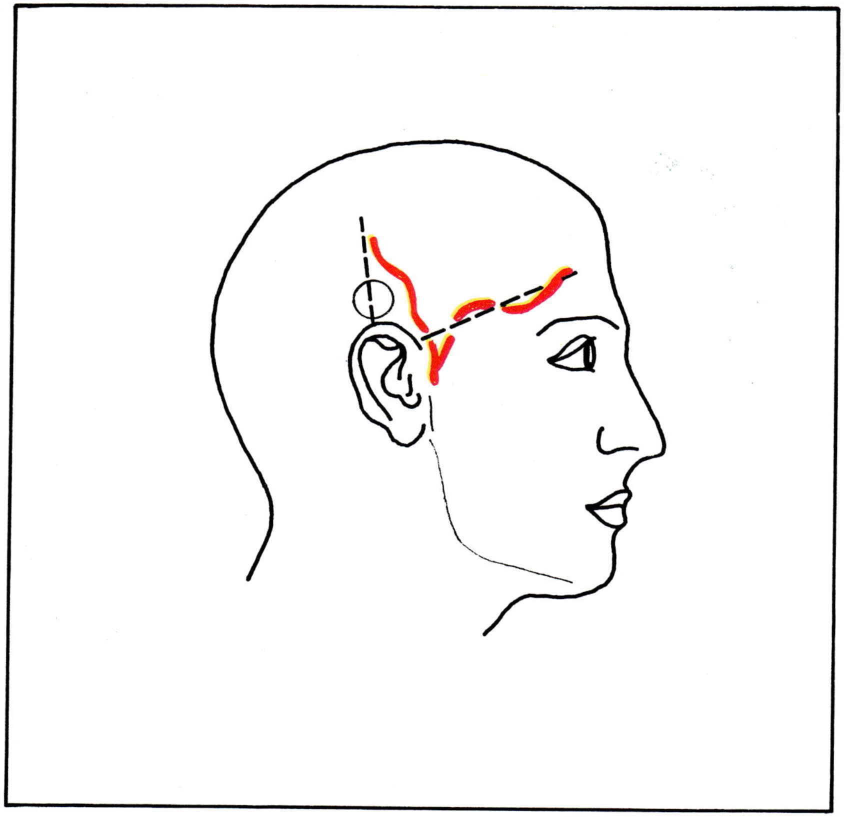

96 When the posterior branch of the superficial temporal artery is unsuitable, its anterior branch or the occipital artery can be mobilised by direct incision and used for anastomosis. In this case a second incision is usually required for placement of the burr hole.

97

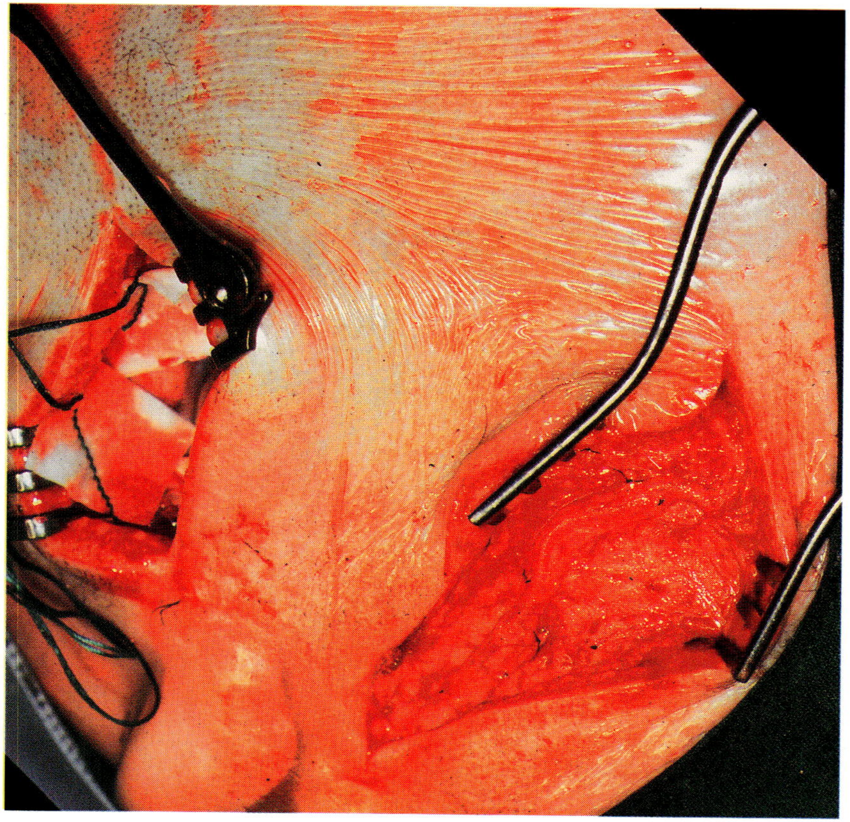

97 The anterior branch of the superficial temporal artery has been mobilised by an incision over it. A burr hole has been made through a supra-auricular incision and a cortical artery of suitable size for anastomosis has been identified.

98

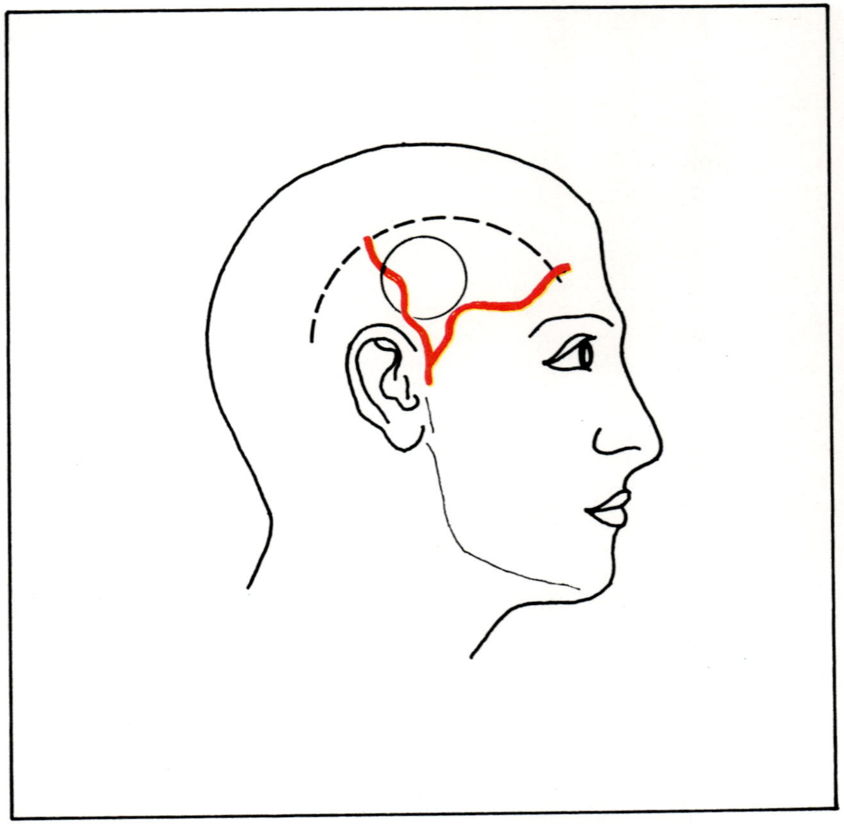

98 Some surgeons prefer to have a larger choice of cortical vessel for anastomosis and a 5 cm to 6 cm disc of bone can be excised. The curved skin incision follows the anterior two-thirds of an arc from the outer margin of the eyebrow to the mastoid process.

99

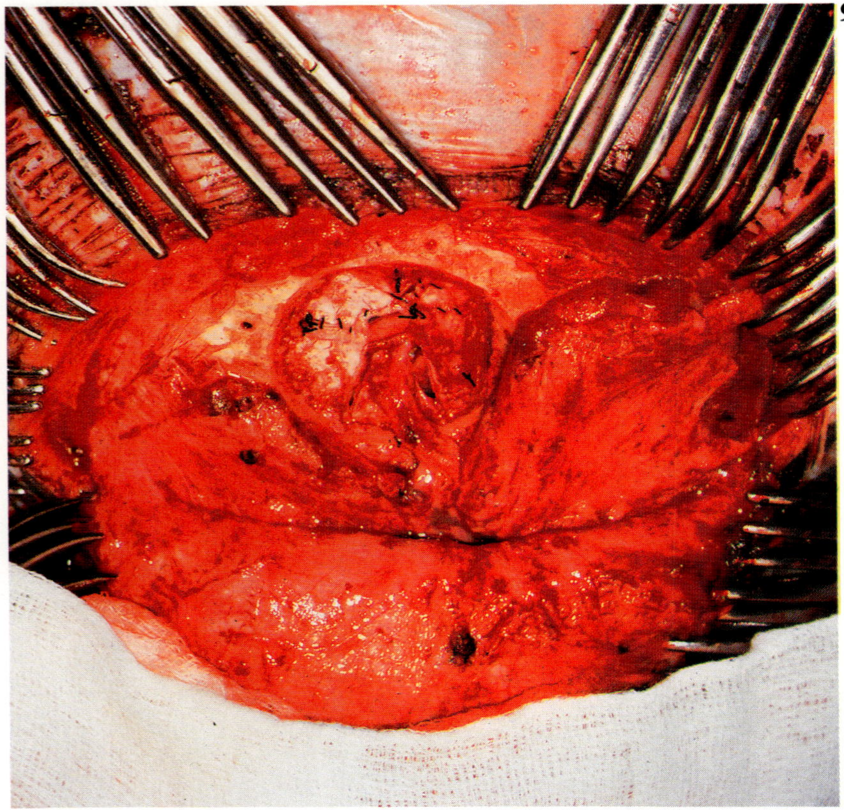

99 The anastomosis between the superficial temporal artery and the cortical branch of the middle cerebral artery has been completed, and dural flaps have been partly sutured together around the bypass artery. An edge of the bony disc will be nibbled away for passage of this vessel and the disc sutured back into position. Suction drainage is usually required.

Postoperative progress

Postoperative progress in these patients is usually uneventful, without the blood pressure instability of carotid endarterectomy. Stitches are removed on the fifth or sixth day and the patients are prescribed anticonvulsive therapy for four to six weeks and longterm antiplatelet medication. Operative stroke morbidity when the procedure has been undertaken for an occluded internal carotid artery in a neurologically stable patient, has been in the region of 1 per cent and longterm stroke morbidity in this high-risk group of patients is low. Transcranial bypass provides a safe addition to stroke prophylaxis surgery; it may also be an alternative to carotid endarterectomy in the high-risk group of patients with bilateral severe internal carotid artery stenosis.

Index

All references are to page numbers